Workbook for

Pharmacy Practice Today for the Pharmacy Technician: Career Training for the Pharmacy Technician

Prepared by:

Marcy May, MEd, CPhT, PhTR
Austin Community College
Austin, TX

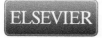

3251 Riverport Lane
St. Louis, Missouri 63043

Workbook for Pharmacy Practice Today for the Pharmacy Technician:
Career Training for the Pharmacy Technician

ISBN: 978-0-323-16987-5

Notices

Knowledge and best practice in this field are constantly changing. As new research and experience broaden our understanding, changes in research methods, professional practices, or medical treatment may become necessary.

Practitioners and researchers must always rely on their own experience and knowledge in evaluating and using any information, methods, compounds, or experiments described herein. In using such information or methods they should be mindful of their own safety and the safety of others, including parties for whom they have a professional responsibility.

With respect to any drug or pharmaceutical products identified, readers are advised to check the most current information provided (i) on procedures featured or (ii) by the manufacturer of each product to be administered, to verify the recommended dose or formula, the method and duration of administration, and contraindications. It is the responsibility of practitioners, relying on their own experience and knowledge of their patients, to make diagnoses, to determine dosages and the best treatment for each individual patient, and to take all appropriate safety precautions.

To the fullest extent of the law, neither the Publisher nor the authors, contributors, or editors, assume any liability for any injury and/or damage to persons or property as a matter of products liability, negligence or otherwise, or from any use or operation of any methods, products, instructions, or ideas contained in the material herein.

Vice President and Publisher: Andrew Allen
Executive Content Strategist: Jennifer Janson
Associate Content Development Specialist: Elizabeth Bawden
Publishing Services Manager: Hemamalini Rajendrababu
Project Manager: Divya Krishnakumar

Working together
to grow libraries in
developing countries

www.elsevier.com • www.bookaid.org

Last digit is the print number: 9 8 7 6 5 4 3 2 1

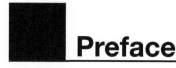

Preface

The goal of this workbook is to help students apply and master key concepts and skills presented in Pharmacy Practice Today for the Pharmacy Technician. The exercises in this workbook will reinforce comprehension of material from the textbook.

The following exercises will provide a sufficient review of concepts and will allow the student to apply the concepts from the text:

- Each chapter begins with a *key term* review. A list of important terms in the corresponding book chapter is provided to test student comprehension of main concepts.
- **Short Answer** response questions apply knowledge learned from the text to a variety of situations.
- A variety of question formats test knowledge of concepts in the book, including **matching, fill-in-the-blank,** and **multiple choice**.
- **Case Thinking** questions provide the practical skills of being a surgical technologist. Patient scenarios allow students to be familiar with real-life situations that will prepare them for the job.
- **Internet Activities** encourage students to research their answer on the internet using trustworthy sources.

Best wishes as you begin your journey to become a pharmacy technician!

Table of Contents

1 Historical Review of Pharmacy Practice

KEY TERMINOLOGY

Provide a definition for each term.

1. Apothecary:

   _____

   _____

2. *Ars medicina:*

   _____

   _____

3. Bodily humors:

   _____

   _____

4. Efficacy:

   _____

   _____

5. Homeostasis:

   _____

   _____

6. Patent medicines:

   _____

   _____

7. Pharmacognosy:

   _____

   _____

8. Pharmacopoeia:

   _____

   _____

9. *Pharmakon*:

_____

_____

10. Toxicology:

_____

_____

11. Wellness:

_____

_____

FILL IN THE BLANK

Complete each statement by providing the word(s) missing where the blank is shown.

1. To be a _____ is to embrace the responsibility of approaching each patient's condition and evaluate how best to restore and sustain health physically, emotionally, and spiritually.

2. Examining the history of both the _____ and _____ of pharmacy practice is key to gaining a sense of purpose and perspective as a patient care provider.

3. _____ _____ must be carefully considered, to render the greatest overall therapeutic benefit.

4. What was evaluated and accepted as concrete truth was often later disproved, as the practice of medicine as an _____ _____ _____ replaced practices that were based on folklore, myth, and mysticism.

5. Patient care providers should be knowledgeable concerning the _____ _____ _____ that is part of many world cultures and how those beliefs influence a patient's ability and desire to be compliant with medical treatment or drug therapy.

6. The Chinese practice of _____ was demonstrated through the use of plant extracts for the treatment of several diseases, and many of these plant extracts have true medicinal value and are still in use today.

7. _____ can be both poison and remedy, depending on the ingredients, their source, and their preparation.

8. Existing drugs in various countries were cataloged by name and used on a central compiled list called a _____.

9. Only since the 1980s or so have pharmacists been more directly involved in making recommendations on the therapeutic appropriateness of various medicines known as _____ _____ _____.

10. Pharmacists traditionally performed all aspects of medication preparation and dispensing, but many of these roles have been assumed by _____ _____.

MATCHING

Match the historical figure with his description.

1. _____ He is referred to as the "father of botany."

2. _____ One of his greatest works is his book *Methodo Medendi*.

3. _____ He is referred to as the "father of medicine."

4. _____ He is referred to as the "father of pharmacognosy."

5. _____ He is referred to as the "Persian Galen."

a. Hippocrates

b. Theophrastus

c. Pedanios Dioscorides

d. Claudius Galen

e. Ibn Sina

MULTIPLE CHOICE

Select the best answer for each question.

1. In the earliest civilizations, illness and disease were attributed to _____.
   a. evidence-based science
   b. evil spirits
   c. homeostasis
   d. body humors

2. One of the most significant finds in ancient Egypt that detailed formulas and remedies was the _____.
   a. *Canon of Medicine*
   b. *material medica*
   c. Ebers Papyrus
   d. *The Great Herbal*

3. The works of _____ greatly influenced Western medicine and are also credited with noting the relationship between emotions and the physical condition.
   a. Hippocrates
   b. Claudius Galen
   c. Emperor Shun-Nung
   d. Ibn Sina

4. The _____ practice of medicine led to an accumulation of practical experience and helped increase an understanding of what is now known as toxicology.
   a. Chinese
   b. Egyptian
   c. Greek
   d. Babylonian

5. The invention of the _____ in 1590 helped identify microorganisms as the cause of disease.
   a. Petri dish
   b. *materia medica*
   c. microscope
   d. pharmacopoeia

6. _____ is an early form of chemistry that involved the process of cooking and combining raw materials into a final preparation.
   a. Toxicology
   b. Pharmacognosy
   c. Pharmakon
   d. Alchemy

7. The first United States Pharmacopoeia (U.S.P.) was published in _____.
   a. 1770
   b. 1820
   c. 1920
   d. 1970

8. In 1804 the state of _____ passed a law requiring a licensing examination for pharmacists wishing to practice their profession.
   a. Louisiana
   b. Massachusetts
   c. Virginia
   d. Georgia

9. Which of the following would *not* be a job responsibility of a pharmacy technician?
   a. Managing inventory
   b. Admixing IVs
   c. Distributing medications
   d. Medication therapy management

10. Only since _____ have pharmacy technicians been subject to a certification examination as a means of determining competence and the attainment of basic subject matter related to their jobs.
    a. 1960
    b. 1975
    c. 1995
    d. 2000

CRITICAL THINKING

Based on what you have learned in the textbook, answer the following questions.

1. How does understanding the history of pharmacy contribute to learning about your role as a pharmacy technician?

   _____

   _____

   _____

2. Even though formal training or education may not be a national requirement, why would it be beneficial to seek and obtain educational training in pharmacy technology?

   _____

   _____

   _____

INTERNET EXERCISES

Answer the following questions by researching your answers on the Internet.

1. Research the type of training you will need to complete to become a pharmacy technician in your state.

   _____

   _____

   _____

2. Many of the medications we still use today were discovered by accident. Some of these medications include aspirin and digitalis. Research each of these naturally occurring products and how they were discovered. What other medications have been discovered from naturally occurring compounds?

   _____

   _____

   _____

3. Complete the research of the scenario proposed in the chapter: Do you have an old family remedy that, although seemingly strange or unscientific, has been an accepted treatment for a particular illness or symptom? Consider some of the ingredients used, and conduct research on the medicinal properties of those components.

   _____

   _____

   _____

2 Pharmacy Law and State Boards of Pharmacy: Examining Regulatory Standards that Govern Pharmacy Practice

KEY TERMINOLOGY

Provide a definition for each term.

1. Administrative (or regulatory) law:

2. Civil liability:

3. Common (or case) law:

4. Criminal liability:

5. Defendant:

6. International law:

7. Law:

8. Legislature:

9. Malfeasance:

10. MSDS:

_____

_____

11. Plaintiff:

_____

_____

12. Statute:

_____

_____

13. Statutory law:

_____

_____

14. Tort:

_____

_____

15. Verdict:

_____

_____

FILL IN THE BLANK

Complete each statement by providing the word(s) missing where the blank is shown.

1. To protect patients, _____ have been established concerning the practice of medicine and the dispensing of pharmaceutical products.

2. Pharmacy practice law has been established in accordance with _____ and _____ laws, so those who practice in the profession must adhere to all applicable laws.

3. Pharmacy laws were designed to shape the day-to-day activities of pharmacists and pharmacy technicians, with the intent to protect the health, welfare, and safety of the _____.

4. Two of the most frequent tasks that technicians perform in _____ practice are processing and filling prescription refills.

5. If a patient requests _____ _____ _____ caps and containers, pharmacy technicians who cashier and dispense these prescriptions must ensure that they educate patients on the risks.

6. Every pharmacy employee should know the location of department _____, as well as hazardous spill kits, eye wash stations, and where to locate all personal protective equipment.

7. Pharmacy technicians must maintain the highest level of moral and ethical conduct and must carefully consider the consequences of _____ federal law.

8. One of the most frequently performed tasks that the community pharmacy technician performs is the processing of third-party claims _____ to insurance companies.

9. Pharmacy technicians must use professional judgment and _____ _____ when speaking to patients to ensure that PHI is not inadvertently disclosed to surrounding patients or customers.

10. Pharmacists and pharmacy technicians must make every effort to _____ situations that could place them in jeopardy of administrative, civil, or criminal liability.

MATCHING

Match each controlled substance with its corresponding DEA controlled substance schedule.

1. _____ phenobarbital

2. _____ carisoprodol

3. _____ oxycodone

4. _____ testosterone

5. _____ morphine

6. _____ cocaine

7. _____ meperidine

8. _____ hydrocodone with acetaminophen

9. _____ diazepam

10. _____ acetaminophen with codeine elixir

a. Schedule I

b. Schedule II

c. Schedule III

d. Schedule IV

e. Schedule V

MULTIPLE CHOICE

Select the best answer for each question.

1. Which of the following is *not* an example of misbranding according to the Food, Drug and Cosmetic Act of 1938?
   a. Using filthy, putrid, or unsanitary substances
   b. Labeling a drug with a treatment claim that is false
   c. Missing directions for use
   d. Missing adequate warnings concerning ingredients that could be habit forming

2. This act further stipulated that prescription drug labels bear the legend "Caution: Federal law prohibits dispensing without a prescription."
   a. The Kefauver-Harris Amendment of 1962
   b. The Poison Prevent Packaging Act of 1970
   c. The Durham-Humphrey Amendment of 1951
   d. The Occupational Safety and Health Act of 1970

3. This amendment to the FDCA expanded the requirement that a drug must be proved to be not only safe but effective as well.
   a. The Kefauver-Harris Amendment of 1962
   b. The Poison Prevention Packing Act of 1970
   c. The Durham-Humphrey Amendment of 1951
   d. The Occupational Safety and Health Act of 1970

4. This act requires the use of child-resistant containers for packaging of most OTC drugs and nearly all prescription drugs.
   a. The Controlled Substance Act
   b. The Poison Prevention Act of 1970
   c. The Kefauver-Harris Amendment of 1962
   d. The Occupational Safety and Health Act of 1970

5. DEA form _____ must be used for a pharmacy to purchase controlled substances.
   a. 41
   b. 106
   c. 222
   d. 224

6. This act created a means to maintain an accurate database of current FDA products that have been assigned an NDC number.
   a. The Orphan Drug Act of 1983
   b. The Drug Price Competition and Patent-Term Restoration Act of 1984
   c. The Prescription Drug Marketing Act of 1987
   d. The Drug Listing Act of 1972

7. This law allows generic drug manufacturers to submit an abbreviated application for new drug approval (ANDA).
   a. The Drug Price Competition and Patent-Term Restoration Act of 1984
   b. The Prescription Drug Marketing Act of 1987
   c. The Drug Listing Act of 1972
   d. The Orphan Drug Act of 1983

8. This law primarily protects patients from receiving dispensed drugs that came from disreputable sources and could be unsafe for use or consumption.
   a. The Drug Price Competition and Patent-Term Restoration Act of 1984
   b. The Prescription Drug Marketing Act of 1987
   c. The Drug Listing Act of 1972
   d. The Orphan Drug Act of 1983

9. Which of the following is not an example of PHI?
   a. Name
   b. Date of birth
   c. Email address
   d. Laboratory results

10. The primary purpose during this drug study phase is to test the drug for efficacy with test subjects that have the disease or clinical symptoms as the drug's intended use.
    a. Phase 1
    b. Phase 2
    c. Phase 3
    d. Phase 4

CRITICAL THINKING

Based on what you have learned in the textbook, answer the following questions.

1. Explain the importance for pharmacy technicians to know and understand the laws that regulate and pertain to pharmacy.

   _____

   _____

   _____

2. While working the in-window at the local community pharmacy, a young woman approaches the window to drop off two new prescriptions to be filled. As you are looking up her patient profile in the computer, she begins to ask questions about her prescription medications and voices that she doesn't understand why she needs to take them. After overhearing the woman's questions, the pharmacist quickly approaches your station and asks "How may I help you?" The woman redirects her questions to the pharmacist, to which the pharmacist replies "Join me at the consultation window to discuss your medications."

   Why do you think the pharmacist intervened when the woman asked her questions? Why did the pharmacist ask the woman to go to the consultation window to answer the questions?

   _____

   _____

   _____

INTERNET EXERCISES

Answer the following questions by researching your answers on the Internet.

1. Research the laws in your state that pertain to pharmacy technician liability. As a pharmacy technician, to what extent could you be held liable? Has reading about the possibility of being held liable for negligence changed your view on always trying your best not to make medication errors?

   _____

   _____

   _____

2. To determine whether a generic drug is bioequivalent, the FDA has developed a listing of therapeutically equivalent drugs in which they designate each drug product with an "A" code or a "B" code. Research what these codes mean and how a drug product's therapeutic code is determined.

_____

_____

_____

3 The Study of Bioethics in Pharmacy Technician Practice

KEY TERMINOLOGY

Provide a definition for each term.

1. Advocacy:

   _____

   _____

2. Autonomy:

   _____

   _____

3. Code:

   _____

   _____

4. Core values:

   _____

   _____

5. Ethical dilemma:

   _____

   _____

6. Ethics:

   _____

   _____

7. Integrity:

   _____

   _____

8. Patient autonomy:

   _____

   _____

FILL IN THE BLANK

Complete each statement by providing the word(s) missing where the blank is shown.

1. The ability to apply _____ or _____ ethical principles appropriately is of great importance in the practice of patient care.

2. Over the centuries, codes have been established that define and express the _____ _____ and _____ of a particular group.

3. The lasting value of good decision making, when exercised for the right reasons, is the development of strong _____ and _____ character.

4. It is up to each _____ _____ to make the choice and commitment to uphold the values of the profession he or she has chosen.

5. When both moral and ethical behavior is demonstrated on a consistent basis, a _____ _____ is set for others in the profession to follow.

6. Pharmacy technicians must always treat patients with respect, in both _____ and _____ communication.

7. Pharmacy technicians must ensure that they consistently collect all the _____ information from a patient.

8. Patients should be treated with _____ and _____, regardless of race, creed, gender, sexual orientation, disease state, demeanor, and the like.

9. Every patient should be given the same degree of attention and _____ _____ _____.

10. Application of the principles of _____, _____ for persons, and _____ by every pharmacy technician will ensure that every patient receives exemplary customer care.

MATCHING

Match each principle from the Code of Ethics for Pharmacy Technicians with its correct description.

1. _____ A pharmacy technician never assists in the dispensing, promoting, or distribution of medications or medical devices that are not of good quality or do not meet the standards required by law.

2. _____ A pharmacy technician respects the confidentiality of patients' records and discloses pertinent information only with proper authorization.

3. _____ A pharmacy technician's first considerations are to ensure the health and safety of the patient and to use knowledge and skills to the best of his or her ability in serving others.

4. _____ A pharmacy technician does not engage in any activity that will discredit the profession, and a pharmacy technician will expose, without fear or favor, illegal or unethical conduct in the profession.

5. _____ A pharmacy technician maintains competency in his or her practice and continually enhances his or her knowledge and expertise.

6. _____ A pharmacy technician supports and promotes honesty and integrity in the profession, which includes a duty to observe the law, maintain the highest moral and ethical conduct at all times, and uphold the ethical principles of the profession.

7. _____ A pharmacy technician associates with and engages in the support of organizations that promote the profession of pharmacy through the utilization and enhancement of pharmacy technicians.

8. _____ A pharmacy technician respects and supports the patient's individuality, dignity, and confidentiality.

9. _____ A pharmacy technician assists and supports the pharmacist in the safe, efficacious, and cost-effective distribution of health services and health care resources.

10. _____ A pharmacy technician respects and values the abilities of pharmacists, colleagues, and other health care professionals.

a. Principle 1

b. Principle 2

c. Principle 3

d. Principle 4

e. Principle 5

f. Principle 6

g. Principle 7

h. Principle 8

i. Principle 9

j. Principle 10

MULTIPLE CHOICE

Select the best answer for each question.

1. Exercising good judgment and ethical behavior requires the application of ethical or _____ to various controversial or seemingly controversial situations.
   a. autonomy
   b. core values
   c. moral principles
   d. advocacy

2. In addition to adhering to the law, pharmacists and pharmacy technicians must also apply _____ when applying the law.
   a. pharmacology
   b. professional judgment
   c. Nuremburg Code
   d. informed consent

3. _____ set forth the expectation that physicians and those involved in the care of human subjects must establish that the medical benefit outweighs any risks involved.
   a. The Hippocratic Oath
   b. The Geneva Convention of Medical Ethics
   c. The Code of Ethics for Pharmacy Technicians
   d. The Declaration of Helsinki

4. _____ is the mechanism that shows respect through patient autonomy.
   a. The Nuremburg Code
   b. Ethics
   c. Informed consent
   d. Conscience

5. Which of the following may influence the development of one's personal definition of ethical or moral behavior?
   a. Religion
   b. Autonomy
   c. Integrity
   d. Codes

6. Which of the following is *not* a key ethical principle to consider when forming a decision for an ethical situation?
   a. Respect for persons
   b. Advocacy
   c. Beneficence
   d. Justice

7. Pharmacy technicians could demonstrate respectful behavior toward a patient by _____.
   a. commenting on a patient's lack of prescription insurance when he or she picks up his or her medications from the pharmacy
   b. yelling across the pharmacy what medications the patient is taking
   c. giving the patient their full focus when communicating with him or her
   d. tapping their feet or standing with arms crossed when a patient is talking to them

8. Why would completing a formal pharmacy technician training program be advantageous?
   a. To gain the valuable knowledge and skills necessary to best serve patients
   b. To have a clear understanding of how to offer focused patient care
   c. To learn the key ethical behaviors pharmacy technicians are expected to demonstrate on a daily basis
   d. All of the above

9. Having _____ will help pharmacy technicians to establish where they stand on various principles in life.
   a. core values
   b. ethical dilemmas
   c. partnerships
   d. shared accountability

10. On which of the following topics must a pharmacy technician stay current and knowledgeable?
    a. State and federal pharmacy laws
    b. Drug doses and dose forms
    c. Licensing and registration requirements
    d. All of the above

CRITICAL THINKING

Based on what you have learned in the textbook, answer the following questions.

1. Why is it important for pharmacy technicians always to have a patient care focus? List a few techniques or reminders for yourself to help you remember and implement them on a daily basis.

   _____

   _____

   _____

2. Using the scenario presented below, apply the five primary steps of the *Framework of Ethical Decision Making* discussed in the chapter. Outline your thoughts and response to the situation. What would you do in this situation? How would you respond?

   John Peterson is a pharmacy technician at a local retail chain store pharmacy. During a busy lunch hour rush, an elderly patient takes several minutes to search through her purse while trying to locate her prescriptions. Visibly annoyed, John snidely inquires of the patient, "Can't you just step aside until you find your prescription? It's busy, and you're holding up the line!"

   _____

   _____

   _____

INTERNET EXERCISES

Answer the following questions by researching your answers on the Internet.

1. Research the Code of Ethics for Pharmacists. Note the uniformity standard across the profession related to the ethical standard of practice for pharmacy technicians.

_____

_____

_____

2. Go to your state's board of pharmacy website and conduct a search of code compliance disciplinary actions that are documented as public record. Note cases that were cited as a consequence of poor professional judgment and the disciplinary action implemented as a result.

_____

_____

_____

Pharmacy Professional Organizations

KEY TERMINOLOGY

Provide a definition for each term.

1. Health literacy:

   _____

   _____

2. White papers:

   _____

   _____

FILL IN THE BLANK

Complete each statement by providing the word(s) missing where the blank is shown.

1. Pharmacy organizations were originally created to provide _____ _____ that would help pharmacists to best protect the health, welfare, and safety of their patients.

2. Many (professional) organizations have sponsored or published research studies, reports, and professional commentaries, sometimes known as _____ _____.

3. The _____ _____ of the Code of Ethics for Pharmacy Technicians is *continuous learning.*

4. Pharmacy technicians should continually seek opportunities to increase their _____ and _____ of how medication is used as well as the technology that helps increase the efficiency and safety of workflow processes.

5. Since the late 1990s, the profession of pharmacy has begun to acknowledge the evolving role of the _____ _____.

6. The need for _____ _____ technicians has been increasingly recognized as a patient safety issue that must be addressed across the nation.

7. Pharmacy technicians should seek out organizations that _____ for technicians and offer opportunities for them to contribute productively to the profession and in a manner that protects the health, safety, and welfare of patients.

8. _____ has contributed universal educational goals and standards for both pharmacy residency and pharmacy technician training programs.

9. The _____ _____ _____ sets a standard for pharmacy technicians to meet and exceed as they proceed through their careers and challenges them to set a higher standard of practice for those to follow in years to come.

10. _____ developed a public advocacy campaign aimed at educating consumers, the health care community, and politicians on the significant contributions that pharmacy technicians make to health care at large.

MATCHING

Match each description with its correct professional pharmacy organization.

1. _____ Was the first professional organization established in the United States

2. _____ Was founded as the second source for pharmacy technicians to gain the CPhT credential by successfully passing its certification examination, the ExCPT

3. _____ Represents what is now the largest component of the pharmacy practice

4. _____ Originated as a hospital pharmacist committee that was part of the Section on Practical Pharmacy and Dispensing

5. _____ Is the largest technician-based national association

6. _____ Began as a networking resource for pharmacy technician educators and has grown into a network of educators from across the United States and Canada

7. _____ Was known as the National Association of Retail Druggists (NARD)

8. _____ Was the first national organization in the United States to offer voluntary pharmacy technician certification

9. _____ Was the first established pharmacy technician association in the United States and was founded in 1979 by volunteer pharmacy technicians

10. _____ The nation's comprehensive resource for pharmaceutical compounding, including raw materials, equipment, technology, education, and professional resources

a. ICPT

b. NCPA

c. ASHP

d. PTCB

e. NACDS

f. APhA

g. PCCA

h. AAPT

i. PTEC

j. NPTA

MULTIPLE CHOICE

Select the best answer for each question.

1. _____ is published by the American Pharmacist Association.
   a. Tech Topics
   b. Pharmacy Today
   c. American Journal of Health-System Pharmacy (AJHP)
   d. *America's Pharmacist Magazine*

2. Which of the following is not a primary goal for ASHP?
   a. Establish minimal standards for the hospital pharmacy practice.
   b. Provide a forum for encouraging the development of new pharmaceutical techniques.
   c. Petition the appropriate legislative and regulatory bodies to serve the needs of those they represent.
   d. Aid the medical profession in extending the economical and rational use of medication.

3. _____ established the *Best Practices for Health-System Pharmacy* to detail standards for those in health-system practice.
   a. PTEC
   b. ICPT
   c. NPTA
   d. ASHP

4. Which of the following organizations is currently the only accrediting body for pharmacy technician training programs?
   a. ASHP
   b. PTCB
   c. AAPT
   d. NPTA

5. The American Society of Health System Pharmacists publishes which of the following professional resources?
   a. *Journal of Pharmacy Technology*
   b. *Tech Trends*
   c. *Handbook on Injectable Drugs*
   d. *America's Pharmacist Magazine*

6. _____ is a nonprofit international organization composed of pharmacy technicians from the United States, Canada, and the United Kingdom.
   a. AAPT
   b. NPTA
   c. ICPT
   d. APhA

7. The Code of Ethics for Pharmacy Technicians is one of the most significant contributions this organization has made.
   a. APhA
   b. NPTA
   c. ASHP
   d. AAPT

8. This organization was the first to offer pharmacy technician-specific continuing education programming during its annual seminar.
   a. NPTA
   b. ASHP
   c. AAPT
   d. PCCA

9. _____ has done much to inspire pharmacy technicians to aspire to higher levels of practice as well as to contribute in more positive ways to their profession.
   a. AAPT
   b. PTCB
   c. NPTA
   d. APhA

10. The primary mission of PTEC is to _____.
    a. help pharmacy technicians "realize their potential" within the profession
    b. promote collaboration among professional pharmacy organizations for the formation and establishment of uniform pharmacy technician education, training, and credentialing standards
    c. offer a credentialing examination to individuals seeking pharmacy technician certification
    d. empower student technicians and certified or registered pharmacy technicians with education and resources to increase their capacity to provide exemplary pharmaceutical services that safeguard the health, welfare, and safety of patients

CRITICAL THINKING

Based on what you have learned in the textbook, answer the following questions.

1. Early pharmacy organizations provided resources to colleges and schools of pharmacy to standardize the education and training of new pharmacists in the United States. Do you think that current pharmacy organizations can and will help achieve the same results for pharmacy technicians? Why or why not? What would be a few benefits for standardized education for pharmacy technicians? How can you help advocate for this?

_____

_____

_____

2. Why is the education of a pharmacy technician never-ending? How could professional pharmacy organizations help with the pursuit of learning new aspects of the profession?

_____

_____

_____

3. If given the opportunity to be more involved with the pharmacy profession, what idea or research would you present at a professional organization's annual meeting?

_____

_____

_____

INTERNET EXERCISES

Answer the following questions by researching your answers on the Internet.

1. Research the pharmacy organizations presented in the chapter. Make a list of resources that are available to nonmembers. What added benefits are there to being a member?

   _____

   _____

   _____

2. Research pharmacy associations for your state. Does your state have one? Does the state association have local chapters? How can you become involved?

   _____

   _____

   _____

3. Research current legislation for pharmacy technicians in your state. What, if any, is currently being discussed for the profession?

   _____

   _____

   _____

5 Medical Terminology: Learning the Language of the Medication Order

KEY TERMINOLOGY

Provide a definition for each term.

1. Combining form:

   _____

   _____

2. Combining vowel:

   _____

   _____

3. Prefix:

   _____

   _____

4. Root:

   _____

   _____

5. Suffix:

   _____

   _____

FILL IN THE BLANK

Complete each statement by providing the word(s) missing where the blank is shown.

1. _____ _____ may be defined as the vocabulary, or *language,* of the practice of medicine.

2. Medical terminology often describes how a physician has directed a patient to take a _____ _____.

3. _____ are translated into a common language that patients should be able to understand and follow concerning how and when to start and stop taking their medication.

4. _____ _____ are responsible for entering prescription data in the community pharmacy practice setting.

5. Interpreting a _____ _____ is much like learning a new language.

6. Learning individual medical terms is simply a matter of putting together the _____ to decode the meaning of the word.

7. The _____ _____ is used when the suffix starts with a consonant.

8. Pharmacy technicians who perform prescription order entry should always consider the _____ _____ of medication administration to ensure patient safety.

9. Pharmacy technicians must carefully review each prescription received from a patient to ensure that the prescriber has noted all necessary information and that the prescription is _____ and _____.

10. Pharmacy technicians must recognize how medical terms are applied in pharmacy practice to preserve the _____, _____, and _____ of patients.

MATCHING

Match each sig code abbreviation with its correct translation.

1. _____ every night   a. QD

2. _____ three times daily   b. BID

3. _____ twice daily   c. TID

4. _____ four times daily   d. QID

5. _____ every day   e. QHS

Match each common medical term to its correct definition.

6. _____ Drugs used to prevent the growth or life of a disease-causing microorganism   a. Angina

7. _____ Abnormal elevation of arterial blood pressure   b. Antibiotics

8. _____ Distress pain (usually in the chest)   c. Carcinogenic

9. _____ Agent that produces cancer   d. Chronic

10. _____ Recurring or ongoing, of varying degrees of severity   e. Hypertension

Match each medical term to its correct translation.

11. _____ Below; deficient or under   a. -algia

12. _____ Slow   b. brady-

13. _____ Process; condition   c. hypo-

14. _____ Within   d. intra-

15. _____ Pain   e. -osis

MULTIPLE CHOICE

Select the best answer for each question.

1. _____ are meant to allow physicians to document medication therapy on a prescription pad more efficiently.
   a. Combining vowel
   b. Medical terms
   c. Abbreviations
   d. Root words

2. The Rx symbol is derived from the Latin word *recipere*, which means _____.
   a. before
   b. to take
   c. write
   d. recipe

3. The word *prescription* literally translates to _____.
   a. to take
   b. write
   c. take thou
   d. written before

4. _____, a regulatory body that accredits hospitals, set forth a list of unapproved abbreviations because of the high risk of misinterpretation or incorrect transcription.
   a. The American Society of Health-System Pharmacists
   b. The Joint Commission
   c. The National Association of Boards of Pharmacy
   d. The Institute for Safe Medicine Practices

5. The central segment, or root, of a word defines _____.
   a. basic anatomical or physical system or structure
   b. number of parts
   c. location, position or direction of movement of an organ or body part
   d. condition, disease, or procedure

6. The first segment, or prefix, of a word will indicate _____.
   a. changes in a word from a noun to an adjective
   b. condition, disease, or procedure
   c. basic anatomical or physical system or structure
   d. time or frequency

7. The last segment, or suffix, of a word will indicate _____.
   a. a reverse meaning of the root
   b. number of parts
   c. a condition, disease, or procedure
   d. a basic anatomical or physical system or structure

8. The most common combining vowel that is used in medical terminology is _____.
   a. -a
   b. -e
   c. -i
   d. -o

9. When forming a term that relates to an anatomical structure, the suffix _____ may be used as a more appropriate ending than a combining vowel.
   a. -ic
   b. -ex
   c. -it
   d. -is

10. A phrase or sentence composed of abbreviated instructions is commonly referred to as _____.
    a. term code
    b. med code
    c. sig code
    d. med terms

CRITICAL THINKING

Based on what you have learned in the textbook, answer the following questions.

1. Why would it be beneficial for a pharmacy technician to have a working knowledge of medical terminology beyond the ability to translate medication orders?

   _____

   _____

   _____

2. Why is it important sometimes to read "between the lines" when translating prescription orders? Give at least two examples of when this should be performed in the pharmacy.

   _____

   _____

   _____

INTERNET EXERCISES

Answer the following questions by researching your answers on the Internet.

1. Research unapproved medication terminology abbreviations on The Joint Commission website. What abbreviations are listed? What is a potential problem with the listed abbreviations? What is suggested as an alternative to avoid potential problems with the listed abbreviations?

_____

_____

_____

2. Research error-prone abbreviations on the Institute for Safe Medication Practices (ISMP) website (www.ismp.org). How do these compare with the abbreviations listed on The Joint Commission "Do Not Use" list?

_____

_____

_____

6 The Structure and Workflow Processes of the Community Pharmacy Practice

KEY TERMINOLOGY

Provide a definition for each term.

1. Adjudication:

   _____

   _____

2. Amber vials:

   _____

   _____

3. Auxiliary labels:

   _____

   _____

4. Counseling area:

   _____

   _____

5. Counting trays:

   _____

   _____

6. Cycle counts:

   _____

   _____

7. Dispense as written (DAW):

   _____

   _____

8. Drug profile:

   _____

   _____

9. Empathy:

_____

_____

10. Inscription:

_____

_____

11. Insurance/payer profile:

_____

_____

12. Medication therapy management:

_____

_____

13. Patient profile:

_____

_____

14. Pharmaceutical elegance:

_____

_____

15. Prescription refill:

_____

_____

16. Production area:

_____

_____

17. Signa:

_____

_____

18. Stock bottle:

_____

_____

19. Superscription:

_____

_____

20. Warning labels:

_____

_____

FILL IN THE BLANK

Complete each statement by providing the word(s) missing where the blank is shown.

1. Pharmacy technicians should gain a sense of the pharmacy's surrounding _____ to better appreciate the types of skills that may be useful in that pharmacy.

2. Before any prescriptions are prepared for dispensing, it is important that the fill area is kept clean and clear to prevent fill errors and to keep from introducing _____ into the products being prepared.

3. Pharmacy staff must work _____ _____ every day to accomplish the variety of tasks associated with the community pharmacy practice.

4. Pharmacy technicians should ensure that they have a clear understanding of how to use all of the _____ of the pharmacy management systems.

5. It is important from an accountability standpoint that the filling technician _____ any prescription he or she has filled.

6. Because of the abuse potential associated with controlled medication, care must be taken to ensure that the prescription is _____ before filling.

7. If a pharmacy technician has any concerns or reservations about a _____, he or she should bring it to the attention of the pharmacist during the order entry, fill, or check processes.

8. If a pharmacy technician knows of a warning or precaution that a patient needs to be aware of, the technician should use that knowledge as a cue to _____ _____ the patient to speak with the pharmacist concerning the medication.

9. The manner in which pharmacy technicians interact with patients during the dispensing process will help to _____ that patient's view of pharmacy services at large.

10. No matter how many times pharmacy technicians hear clinical information being disseminated, it is not _____ _____ for them to provide that information themselves.

MATCHING

Match each duty in the pharmacy with the person who is designated to perform it.

1. _____ Stock medication on shelves

2. _____ Verify order entry accuracy against the written prescription for a final check

3. _____ Accept a verbal order for a new prescription from a patient care provider

4. _____ Control the inventory of medication

5. _____ Read back instructions as printed on the prescription label

6. _____ Encourage patients to seek out the pharmacist for counseling

7. _____ Counsel patient on the use of the medication

8. _____ Administer oral or injectable immunizations after required training

9. _____ Enter prescriptions into the computerized order entry system

10. _____ Verify the patient's prescription benefit eligibility

a. Pharmacy technician

b. Pharmacist

MULTIPLE CHOICE

Select the best answer for each question.

1. Chain and community pharmacies may offer which of the following services to the public?
   a. Immunizations
   b. Homeopathic and alternative medication therapy
   c. Home health medical equipment
   d. All of the above

2. Which of the following actions will take place at the front counter prescription drop-off area?
   a. Prescription order entry
   b. Drug selection
   c. Dispensing and accepting payment from patient
   d. Medication preparation, packaging, and labeling

3. Final check by the pharmacist of medications being dispensed will likely take place at this workstation in the pharmacy.
   a. Front counter prescription drop-off area
   b. Medication storage areas
   c. Production area
   d. Patient counseling area

4. One of the most important interactions in the community pharmacy settings is the initial conversation between the pharmacy technician and a new patient during this stage of processing a prescription.
   a. Stage 1
   b. Stage 2
   c. Stage 3
   d. Stage 4

5. Controlled medications that fall in DEA schedules III through V may be refilled up to _____ times.
   a. 2
   b. 3
   c. 5
   d. 6

6. Drug information about the drug product that prints along with the dispensing label and is given to the patient during the prescription dispensing process is often referred to as a _____.
   a. drug monograph
   b. national drug code
   c. drug facts
   d. drug profile

7. When selecting a drug from the pharmacy drug storage area to be dispensed, which of the following should be performed to ensure the correct drug from the stock area was pulled?
   a. Check the NDC number of the drug pulled.
   b. Check the drug pulled against the hard copy prescription.
   c. Check the drug pulled against the prescription label.
   d. All of the above

8. Which of the following does *not* need to be on a retail prescription label?
   a. Pharmacy name, address, and phone number
   b. Directions for use
   c. Date prescription written
   d. Prescriber name

9. The _____ requires that childproof caps be placed on dispensing containers unless a patient specifically requires non-childproof lids.
   a. Controlled Substance Act
   b. Poison Prevention Act of 1970
   c. Kefauver-Harris Amendment of 1962
   d. Occupational Safety and Health Act of 1970

10. What would likely be the last digit of the DEA number for Dr. Jones if it was AJ258455 _____?
    a. 0
    b. 1
    c. 3
    d. 9

CRITICAL THINKING

Based on what you have learned in the textbook, answer the following questions.

1. How does the location of the community pharmacy influence the variety of medications available for dispensing in the pharmacy and on the OTC shelves?

   _____

   _____

   _____

2. Explain the importance of always asking a patient whether he or she is taking any other medications, including OTC medicines, vitamins, and herbal or alternative medicinal products every time he or she fills a prescription at the pharmacy.

   _____

   _____

   _____

INTERNET EXERCISES

Answer the following questions by researching your answers on the Internet.

1. Not all prescription medication requires a childproof cap on dispensing containers. Research which drugs are exempt from the Poison Prevention Act of 1970 and list what they are.

   _____

   _____

   _____

2. The DEA categorizes controlled medications into five schedules. Research the drugs that are designated as a controlled substance and list at least two drugs from each schedule.

   _____

   _____

   _____

7 Team Building and Professionalism in Pharmacy Practice: How Pharmacists and Technicians Collaborate to Foster a Multidisciplinary Mindset

KEY TERMINOLOGY

Provide a definition for each term.

1. Collaboration:

_____

_____

2. Multidisciplinary mindset:

_____

_____

3. Soft skills:

_____

_____

4. Time management:

_____

_____

5. Workflow management:

_____

_____

FILL IN THE BLANK

Complete each statement by providing the word(s) missing where the blank is shown.

1. A critical element of _____ in the health care environment is the development of a patient focus.

2. The physical appearance of a pharmacy technician is a critical factor for projecting an image of professionalism that will reflect _____ on one's employer and the profession in general.

3. Recognizing one's role as part of a greater _____ should serve as a greater motivator to achieve higher-quality results.

4. One should ask questions related to the skills and experience that each pharmacy _____ _____ possesses, so that a new technician will know whose expertise to seek out in given situations.

5. A technician's ability to shift and function in a _____ of settings will be more useful to an employer in terms of job retention.

6. Technicians may stay fresh and _____ by seeking ways to continue to develop themselves professionally.

7. Healthy and productive workplace _____ make it possible for a pharmacy to provide patient care through the management of pharmacy workflow.

8. The driving force behind people who take responsibility for their own _____ and the quality of work they produce is accountability.

9. Assisting and supporting the pharmacists means that technicians should perform their job in a way that allows the pharmacists to better serve _____.

10. Every member of the health care team is _____ and needed, and each member must know his or her role, legal responsibilities, and scope of practice.

MATCHING

Match each soft skill with its corresponding definition.

1. _____ An individual's sense of duty or obligation to a commitment or expectation

2. _____ The identification of factors in a situation that may drive a person to action without prompting

3. _____ Use of a step-by-step (systematic) approach when taking action, in light of possible variables

4. _____ A personal attitude or perspective that focuses primarily on the most desirable or positive aspects of a person, place, or situation

5. _____ The ability to identify with another person's perspective or recognize the value of another person's perspective

6. _____ Firm adherence to a code of moral values; the quality or state of being complete or undivided

7. _____ A subjective means of evaluating a situation in terms of its humorous or comedic context

8. _____ The ability to apply practicality to a situation, based on factors that are commonly known, visible, or easily identifiable

9. _____ Often defined by cultural traditions or social trends, the most appropriate manner in which to treat other individuals or approach a given situation

10. _____ Proficient demonstration of sending and receiving information by using verbal, nonverbal, written, and electronic forms of communication

11. _____ A combination of behaviors that allows individuals to make the overall best use of their time

a. Common sense

b. Motivation/initiative

c. Integrity

d. Time management

e. Optimism

f. Good manners/social skills

g. Accountability

h. Empathy

i. Sense of humor

j. Critical thinking

k. Effective communication

MULTIPLE CHOICE

Select the best answer for each question.

1. Inappropriate professional attire would include:
   a. Slacks and button-up shirt
   b. Comfortable, close-toed shoes
   c. Conservative use of jewelry and cosmetics
   d. Jeans and flip-flops

2. Not asking to take a lunch break right in the middle of a busy time of day would demonstrate which of the following soft skills?
   a. Sense of humor
   b. Integrity
   c. Common sense
   d. Social skills

3. Saying "please" and "thank you" is an example of using this soft skill.
   a. Accountability
   b. Good manners
   c. Common sense
   d. Integrity

4. Turning in money or credit cards left behind by a patient is a good example of demonstrating _____.
   a. Optimism
   b. Empathy
   c. Integrity
   d. Time management

5. The ability to validate a patient's concern or emotional response by identifying with his or her perspective demonstrates this soft skill.
   a. Integrity
   b. Sense of humor
   c. Common sense
   d. Empathy

6. Spending time on the most important work and completing it in an efficient manner would demonstrate this soft skill.
   a. Empathy
   b. Sense of humor
   c. Time management
   d. Social skills

7. If you are able to view the glass as "half-full" and tend to focus on the strengths of others rather than shortcomings, you have this soft skill.
   a. Optimism
   b. Empathy
   c. Sense of humor
   d. Time management

8. Pharmacy technicians may begin the process of building successful workplace relationships by doing which of the following?
   a. Developing a team-oriented mindset
   b. Learning the personalities of co-workers
   c. Conducting a personal inventory of one's strengths and weaknesses
   d. All of the above

9. New technicians should avoid this behavior, which can place them at odds with their co-workers and hinder workplace relationships.
   a. Participating in workplace gossip
   b. Expressing resistance to helping others or waiting to be asked to do so
   c. Arriving early to work and staying until the end of the scheduled time
   d. Taking oneself lightly

10. Which of the following processes must be performed according to established guidelines?
    a. Aseptic IV admixture
    b. Batch processing
    c. Processing a prescription
    d. All of the above

CRITICAL THINKING

Based on what you have learned in the textbook, answer the following questions.

1. It is 8:55 on Friday night. You are busily working to finish up your tasks for the day so you can go home on time when the pharmacy closes at 9 pm. An elderly gentleman you do not recognize approaches the intake window to have his antiseizure prescription refilled. On inspection of his prescription bottle, you notice it is from another pharmacy you know that is already closed for the evening. Use the five steps to problem solving to solve this problem.

_____

_____

_____

2. Using the scenario from the previous question, what soft skills can the pharmacy technician demonstrate by helping solve the problem?

_____

_____

_____

INTERNET EXERCISES

Answer the following questions by researching your answers on the Internet.

1. Research local pharmacies in your area, and read the mission statements on their websites. After reading various mission statements, determine which mission statement best aligns with what your mission statement would be. Would this pharmacy be a place you could see yourself working in?

_____

_____

_____

2. Time management does not always come easy. Research tips on how better to manage your time. Are these tips something you would be able to incorporate into your personal and work time?

_____

_____

_____

8 Pharmacology: The Study of Drugs and Their Effects

KEY TERMINOLOGY

Provide a definition for each term.

1. Absorption:

_____

_____

2. Bioavailability:

_____

_____

3. Biotransformation:

_____

_____

4. Distribution:

_____

_____

5. Dosing schedule:

_____

_____

6. Drug:

_____

_____

7. Drug delivery system:

_____

_____

8. Duration of action:

_____

_____

9. Efficacy:

_____

_____

10. Enteral:

_____

_____

11. Homeopathic medicine:

_____

_____

12. Hydrophilic:

_____

_____

13. Hydrophobic:

_____

_____

14. Legend drug:

_____

_____

15. Metabolism:

_____

_____

16. Metabolite:

_____

_____

17. Onset of action:

_____

_____

18. Parenteral:

_____

_____

19. Pathophysiology:

_____

_____

20. Pharmacognosy:

_____

_____

21. Pharmacokinetics:

_____

_____

22. Pharmacology:

_____

_____

23. Physiology:

_____

_____

24. Toxicology:

_____

_____

FILL IN THE BLANK

Complete each statement by providing the word(s) missing where the blank is shown.

1. A working knowledge of the clinical basis of _____ _____ improves the technician's ability to help the pharmacist safely and effectively provide pharmaceutical care to patients.

2. Drugs are derived from _____ or _____ sources.

3. All matter tends to flow naturally from an area of higher concentration into an area of lower concentration to create a balance, or _____.

4. _____ _____ allows a drug to be transported across the plasma cell membrane regardless of the drug concentration.

5. The greater the concentration of protein-binding drug in the bloodstream, the fewer the number of unbound free drug molecules for _____.

6. _____ drugs bind to the receptor site and perform their intended action either by activating a receptor that had been in a resting state or by turning off a receptor that had been activated.

7. _____ drugs bind to receptor sites to block or prevent another drug or natural body chemical from binding to or activating the receptor site.

8. The body's response to a drug is linked to the amount and _____ of the dose administered in several ways.

9. The _____ system is the emergency system that creates the "fight or flight" response.

10. The _____ system is the dominant controller of autonomic systems, particularly during times of "rest and digest."

MATCHING

Match each pregnancy category with its correct description.

1. _____ These drugs have not undergone clinical trials, or no data are available on their use in humans during pregnancy; therefore, the therapeutic benefits must be carefully weighed against the possible risk.

2. _____ These drugs have been tested and have proved to be safe for administration.

3. _____ These drugs have been clinically proven to cause birth defects and *must not* be used during pregnancy.

4. _____ These drugs have been tested in the laboratory, but their safety in humans has not been fully validated.

a. Category A

b. Category B

c. Category C

d. Category X

MULTIPLE CHOICE

Select the best answer for each question.

1. _____ is the process by which natural or biopharmaceutical products are administered to diagnose, treat, cure, prevent, or mitigate disease.
   a. Passive transport
   b. Drug concentration
   c. Medication therapy
   d. Plasma binding

2. Which of the following elements may not be specified on a prescription or medication order?
   a. Product name
   b. Duration of therapy
   c. Route of administration
   d. Duration of action

3. _____ can affect the absorption of a drug.
   a. Drug pH
   b. Product name
   c. Distribution
   d. First-pass effect

4. Which of the following patient-specific factors may affect the storage of hydrophobic drugs?
   a. Age
   b. Obesity
   c. Disease state
   d. Psychological factors

5. Metabolism usually takes place in the liver, but it also may occur in the intestines, lungs, kidneys, or other cellular structures with the assistance of _____.
   a. agonists
   b. perspiration
   c. saliva
   d. enzymes

6. _____ are unexpected adverse drug reactions that indicate the need for an alternate form of drug therapy.
   a. Desensitization
   b. Idiosyncratic reactions
   c. Side effects
   d. Adverse events

7. Skeletal muscle movement occurs when the neurotransmitter _____ activates communication between nerve cells and muscle cells.
   a. interferon
   b. epinephrine
   c. acetylcholine
   d. norepinephrine

8. Drugs used to treat common diseases of the musculoskeletal system may include _____.
   a. glucosteroids
   b. benzodiazepines
   c. catecholamines
   d. beta-blockers

9. When dispensing GI medication, which of the following auxiliary labels may be affixed to the dispensing container to ensure the medication's therapeutic effect is achieved?
   a. Avoid antacids, dairy, and iron products before and after taking.
   b. Avoid alcohol.
   c. Shake well.
   d. All of the above

10. The hormone _____ is essential to the regulation of carbohydrates, fat, and protein metabolism and enables glucose to be carried out of the bloodstream and used in various cells.
   a. prolactin
   b. insulin
   c. calcitonin
   d. glucagon

CRITICAL THINKING

Based on what you have learned in the textbook, answer the following questions.

1. As a pharmacy technician, why is it important to understand the function of medications and their effects on the body?

   _____

   _____

   _____

2. Why it is important to place the proper auxiliary or warning labels on medications dispensed from the pharmacy and to bring these labels to the attention of the patient?

   _____

   _____

   _____

INTERNET EXERCISES

Answer the following questions by researching your answers on the Internet.

1. Foods that contain tyramine can be dangerous to a patient's blood pressure when the patient is taking drugs that are part of the monoamine oxidase inhibitor (MAOI) drug class. Research which drugs are part of the MAOI drug class. How can knowing what these drugs are help you in practice?

   _____

   _____

   _____

2. Many drugs can be used to treat various conditions and diseases. It is sometimes not easy to remember every detail of every drug available. Research online resources that are available to help answer questions about specific medications. How can these resources be helpful in practice?

   _____

   _____

   _____

9 Introduction to Pharmaceutical Dosage Forms

KEY TERMINOLOGY

Provide a definition for each term.

1. Buccal:

_____

_____

2. Dosage form:

_____

_____

3. Drug metabolism:

_____

_____

4. Local effect:

_____

_____

5. Parenteral:

_____

_____

6. Pharmacokinetics:

_____

_____

7. Sublingual:

_____

_____

8. Systemic effect:

_____

_____

9. Troche:

_____

_____

FILL IN THE BLANK

Complete each statement by providing the word(s) missing where the blank is shown.

1. The term _____ _____ _____ also refers to the physical and chemical properties of the drug and how it will affect the patient.

2. An aspect of medication therapy management is ensuring that a patient receives the most appropriate _____.

3. Drugs that elicit an external response have _____ _____.

4. Drugs that must be transported via the bloodstream and metabolized (broken down and converted) into cellular building blocks by the liver or other systems elicit _____ _____.

5. Oral _____ _____ are the most commonly dispensed drug dosage form.

6. A drug's _____ _____ influences how the active ingredient takes action in the body.

7. Patients should be cautioned that chewing an extended-release drug can have _____ _____.

8. _____ are manufactured with either a soft or hard shell.

9. _____ are manufactured using absorption bases that are either solid or semisolid at room temperature.

10. Because they generally require some instrument of measurement, _____ may not always be the most convenient drug delivery system.

MATCHING

Using the following image, match each route of administration with the correct description.

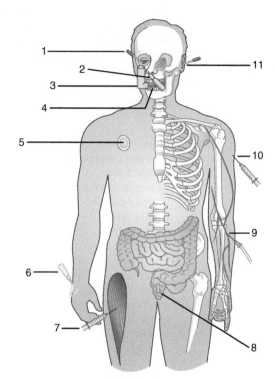

1. _____

2. _____

3. _____

4. _____

5. _____

6. _____

7. _____

8. _____

9. _____

10. _____

11. _____

a. Otic

b. Ocular

c. Sublingual

d. Transdermal

e. Subcutaneous

f. Nasal

g. Suppository

h. Intramuscular

i. Oral

j. Intravenous

k. Topical

MULTIPLE CHOICE

Select the best answer for each question.

1. A drug delivery system refers to all of the following *except* _____.
   a. a physical device used to administer a drug
   b. a drug's active ingredient
   c. a physical characteristic of a drug that affects the way the body breaks down the drug
   d. a means by which a drug is delivered into the body

2. Which of the following would have faster absorption?
   a. Oral tablet
   b. Oral suspension
   c. Oral capsule
   d. IV liquid

3. _____ must be ingested and then broken down in the stomach or intestines before transport to the liver for metabolism.
   a. Cream
   b. Oral liquid
   c. Oral tablet
   d. Sublingual tablet

4. _____ are the most common oral solid dosage forms for medication.
   a. Tablets
   b. Capsules
   c. Powders
   d. Granules

5. A(n) _____ breaks down in the stomach for absorption and transport for metabolism and generally takes effect quickly and does not remain in the bloodstream for an extended period.
   a. sustained-release drug
   b. fast-dissolving drug
   c. extended-release drug
   d. immediate-release drug

6. A(n) _____ is ideal for the treatment of chronic conditions because it is designed to break down more gradually to allow for uniform absorption of the drug in the GI tract over an extended period.
   a. fast-dissolving drug
   b. extended-release drug
   c. immediate-release drug
   d. enteric-coated drug

7. Many over-the-counter antacids and combination cold and flu products are manufactured in this dosage form.
   a. Suppositories
   b. Bulk powders
   c. Granules
   d. Capsules

8. The semisolid dosage form may be administered by all of the following routes of administration *except* the _____.
   a. intravenous route
   b. ocular route
   c. nasal route
   d. vaginal route

9. These products are very thick so that they can remain on the surface of the skin to act as a barrier; they are not absorbed.
   a. Emulsions
   b. Lubricants
   c. Emollients
   d. Pastes

10. This is one of the most common routes of parenteral administration.
   a. Intrathecal
   b. Intramuscular
   c. Intrasynovial
   d. Intraarticular

CRITICAL THINKING

Based on what you have learned in the textbook, answer the following questions.

1. Why is it important for pharmacy technicians to be knowledgeable about the most therapeutically appropriate use of drug delivery systems? How can this reduce medication errors?

   _____

   _____

   _____

2. List at least one advantage and one disadvantage of solid dosage forms, semisolid dosage forms, and liquid dosage forms that were not discussed in the chapter.

_____

_____

_____

INTERNET EXERCISES

Answer the following questions by researching your answers on the Internet.

1. A disadvantage of liquid dosage forms is the storage requirements because some liquid medications require refrigeration. Research storage requirements for liquid medications. List at least two medications that are available in liquid dosage forms that should be refrigerated.

_____

_____

_____

2. As discussed in the chapter, extended-release dosage forms allow for uniform absorption of the drug over an extended period of time, and this makes them ideal for chronic conditions. Research medications that are available in an extended-release dose form. List two extended-release medications and the chronic conditions they are intended to treat.

_____

_____

_____

10 Pharmaceutical Calculations

Provide a definition for each term.

1. AWP:

_____

_____

2. Fraction:

_____

_____

3. Gross profit:

_____

_____

4. Improper fraction:

_____

_____

5. Markup:

_____

_____

6. Markup rate:

_____

_____

7. Mixed fraction:

_____

_____

8. Net profit:

_____

_____

9. Overhead:

_____

_____

10. Proper fraction:

_____

_____

11. Proportion:

_____

_____

12. Ratio:

_____

_____

FILL IN THE BLANK

Complete each statement by providing the word(s) missing where the blank is shown.

1. The ability to perform a calculation or measure a dose accurately directly affects patients' _____ and _____.

2. _____ and _____ compounding generally require the calculation of dosages or quantities.

3. Pharmacy technicians must continually work to improve their skill, accuracy, and confidence in pharmaceutical _____ _____.

4. Most pharmacy math calculations can be solved if the technician knows how to set up the problem or equation _____.

5. A fraction is composed of two parts, the _____ (number of parts) and the _____ (how many parts to make a whole).

6. Fractions and decimals are commonly written as _____ to describe the strength of a medication.

7. Most dosage calculations performed by pharmacy technicians can be done using the _____ calculation method.

8. The _____ system of measurement is used most frequently in both community and hospital pharmacies.

9. For prescription purposes, time is written in _____ time to help prevent confusion and time misinterpretation.

10. The most accurate way to determine the strength of a child's dose based on the adult dose is to use the _____ _____ _____ rule.

MATCHING

Match each metric measurement with its corresponding equivalent.

1. _____ 1 grain   a. 5 mL

2. _____ 1 milligram   b. 65 mg

3. _____ 1 pound   c. 1000 g

4. _____ 1 kilogram   d. 1000 mg

5. _____ 1 liter   e. 1000 mcg

6. _____ 1 teaspoon   f. 1000 mL

7. _____ 1 gram   g. 454 g

8. _____ 1 gallon   h. 15 mL

9. _____ 1 tablespoon   i. 473 mL

10. _____ 1 pint   j. 3785 mL

MULTIPLE CHOICE

Select the best answer for each question.

1. Convert 24 to a Roman numeral.
   a. VVIX
   b. XXIV
   c. XXVI
   d. VVXI

2. Convert XLIV to an Arabic numeral.
   a. 26
   b. 94
   c. 14
   d. 44

3. Convert 8:30 pm to military time.
   a. 0830
   b. 1830
   c. 2030
   d. 2230

4. Convert 78°F to °C.
   a. 25.6°C
   b. 61.1°C
   c. 108.4°C
   d. 172.4°C

5. If a patient takes 2 capsules of a certain medication, he will receive 200 mg of the active ingredient. If the patient is prescribed to take 2 capsules twice daily, how much total active ingredient will he be receiving in 5 days?
   a. 2000 mcg
   b. 2 g
   c. 1000 mcg
   d. 1 g

6. Amoxicillin 250 mg/5 mL is prescribed. The dosage is 1 teaspoon per dose two times a day. How much amoxicillin will be taken if a 10-day regimen is prescribed?
   a. 2500 mg
   b. 2.5 g
   c. 5 g
   d. 5000 g

7. A prescription calls for ibuprofen 600 mg to be given three times a day for 5 days. If ibuprofen 600 mg tablets are available, how many tablets should be given to complete the order?
   a. 15 tablets
   b. 5 tablets
   c. 10 tablets
   d. 30 tablets

8. A prescription calls for amoxil 125 mg/5 mL liquid. The directions state to take 125 mg twice daily for 10 days. How much of the medication should be dispensed?
   a. 5 mL
   b. 100 mg
   c. 50 mL
   d. 100 mL

9. How many milligrams of hydrocortisone are needed to prepare 1000 g of a 1% hydrocortisone cream?
   a. 10 mg
   b. 10,000 mg
   c. 1 mg
   d. 100 mg

10. A 60-g tube of cream costs the pharmacy $23.60. The pharmacy adds an 8% markup. What is the selling price of the tube of cream?
   a. $1.89
   b. $21.71
   c. $44.56
   d. $25.49

CRITICAL THINKING

Based on what you have learned in the textbook, answer the following questions.

1. A patient receives 2 L of IV fluid at 100 mL/hour that starts at midnight. At what time will this IV run out?

_____

_____

_____

2. How many liters of IV fluid will be delivered over 24 hours if it is set to infuse 20 drops/mL at 40 drops/min?

_____

_____

_____

3. The doctor has prescribed 2% hydrocortisone cream. The tube available in your pharmacy does not have a percentage strength printed on it, but it does tell you that each gram of cream contains 20 mg of drug. Is this the right percent strength?

_____

_____

_____

INTERNET EXERCISES

Answer the following questions by researching your answers on the Internet.

1. Temperature affects the physical and chemical stability of medications. A critical task of the pharmacy technician is to check and log refrigerator temperatures to ensure that products in the refrigerator are stored within the appropriate temperature range. Research what may happen when medications that should be refrigerated are stored at room temperature. How can improper storage affect the medication? Why is it important to store medications at the proper temperature?

_____

_____

_____

2. Research body surface area (BSA). What other methods are available to determine BSA besides using a nomogram as discussed in the chapter?

_____

_____

_____

11 The Principles of Nonsterile Pharmaceutical Compounding

KEY TERMINOLOGY

Provide a definition for each term.

1. Aromatic waters:

   _____

   _____

2. Class A balance:

   _____

   _____

3. Compounding slab:

   _____

   _____

4. Conical graduates:

   _____

   _____

5. Counter balance:

   _____

   _____

6. Cylindrical graduates:

   _____

   _____

7. Dispersions:

   _____

   _____

8. Electronic balance:

   _____

   _____

9. Elixirs:

   _____

   _____

10. Emulsion:

   _____

   _____

11. Extracts:

   _____

   _____

12. Fluid extract:

   _____

   _____

13. Geometric dilution:

   _____

   _____

14. Homogenous:

   _____

   _____

15. Irrigations:

   _____

   _____

16. Levigate:

   _____

   _____

17. Meniscus:

   _____

   _____

18. Mortar:

   _____

   _____

19. Ointment:

   _____

   _____

20. Paste:

   _____

   _____

21. Pestle:

_____

_____

22. Solution:

_____

_____

23. Solvent:

_____

_____

24. Spirits:

_____

_____

25. Syrups:

_____

_____

26. Tinctures:

_____

_____

27. Triturate:

_____

_____

FILL IN THE BLANK

Complete each statement by providing the word(s) missing where the blank is shown.

1. _____ _____ is the art of mixing raw materials with active drug substances to create a drug product that can be dispensed to the patient.

2. Compounding pharmacies create opportunities for health care providers to prescribe medications in dosage forms that best suit _____ _____.

3. To ensure that the patient receives the right dose, a pharmacy technician must calculate _____ and then _____ the right amount of the right ingredients.

4. Many _____ dosage forms may be prepared for a patient by using commercially prepared drugs and raw materials.

5. During the compounding process, if a tablet has a coating, _____ _____ to verify that the correct product was selected.

6. The compounding pharmacist must ensure continued _____ and _____ stability and a final product that satisfies the patient's needs.

7. Pharmacy technicians must have a working knowledge of common _____ _____ _____ that may be used and also must know how to _____ among various systems of measurement.

8. Solid drugs are measured by _____, and a balance must be used to measure the solid drug or other compound.

9. Liquid measurement devices are _____ to reflect units of volume.

10. Every compounding process should begin with proper _____ _____ with an antiseptic product that can kill bacteria on the surface of the hands.

MATCHING

Match each component of the product label with its correct label.

1. _____
2. _____
3. _____
4. _____
5. _____

1. ─┤**Drug Product 20 mg/5 mL**

Shake Well

Protect from Light

2. ─┤Store in Refrigerator

3. ─┤MM

Exp: 10/31/11 ├─ 5.

Lot: C10012011001 ├─ 4.

a. Storage requirements

b. Name of the preparation

c. Initials of the compounder

d. Beyond-use date

e. Internal lot number

MULTIPLE CHOICE

Select the best answer for each question.

1. Compounding pharmacies typically provide products and services to patients and customers who _____.
   a. need formulations not typically produced by drug manufacturers
   b. need a customized dosage form
   c. are seeking homeopathic, naturopathic, and other alternative medications
   d. All of the above

2. A recognized source of information for compounding professionals is _____.
   a. FDA
   b. PCCA
   c. USP
   d. NF

3. Individuals involved in the compounding of nonsterile pharmaceuticals must observe regulatory standards established by the _____.
   a. FDA
   b. PCCA
   c. USP
   d. NF

4. What type of measuring device should be used when measuring a volatile liquid ingredient?
   a. Plastic
   b. Glass
   c. Porcelain
   d. Brass

5. When preparing a nonsterile pharmaceutical compound, a _____ is used to crush solids.
   a. mortar and pestle
   b. spatula
   c. homogenizer
   d. compounding slab

6. A _____ is vital to ensuring that the patient knows the time frame in which a product may be safely administered and considered physically, chemically, and therapeutically stable.
   a. master record formula
   b. lot number
   c. preparation name
   d. beyond-use date

7. Water-containing formulations that are prepared from ingredients in solid form should have an auxiliary label of _____.
   a. Store in refrigerator.
   b. Store in dry place.
   c. Store in freezer.
   d. Store at room temperature.

8. When compounding a solid nonaqueous drug preparation with an active ingredient that is a USP/NF substance, the maximum beyond-use date should be _____.
   a. 14 days
   b. 30 days
   c. 6 months
   d. 1 year

9. Only when _____ measures have been applied can the compounded drug preparation effectiveness be assessed.
   a. quality control
   b. quality assurance
   c. acceptable volume/weight
   d. equipment

10. USP Chapter _____ details the regulatory standards for nonsterile pharmaceutical compounding.
    a. 71
    b. 85
    c. 795
    d. 797

CRITICAL THINKING

Based on what you have learned in the textbook, answer the following questions.

1. Why would it be beneficial to learn the art of extemporaneous (nonsterile) compounding?

_____

_____

_____

2. Why is there a growing need for pharmaceutical compounding services? How can a compounding pharmacy meet this growing need?

_____

_____

_____

3. You are to make 120 mL of baclofen 5 mg/mL using the following formula:

Baclofen 5 mg/mL

Baclofen 20-mg tablets	15 tablets
Glycerin	qs
Syrup	qsad 60 mL

How much of each ingredient will be needed? What should the beyond-use date be?

_____

_____

_____

INTERNET EXERCISES

Answer the following questions by researching your answers on the Internet.

1. Research PCCA. What resources are available to support compounding pharmacies?

   _____

   _____

   _____

2. Research the compounding laws in your state for pharmacy technicians. Do you need additional or special training to perform extemporaneous compounding? Do you need additional continuing education?

   _____

   _____

   _____

3. Research extemporaneous compounding certifications. Where could you obtain specialized training? What would be the cost? Do you think you would be interested in pursuing this to enhance your skills?

   _____

   _____

   _____

12 Pharmacy Billing and Claims Processing

KEY TERMINOLOGY

Provide a definition for each term.

1. Beneficiary:

   _____

   _____

2. Claim:

   _____

   _____

3. Co-insurance:

   _____

   _____

4. Co-pay:

   _____

   _____

5. Deductible:

   _____

   _____

6. Medicare:

   _____

   _____

7. Preexisting condition:

   _____

   _____

8. Premium:

   _____

   _____

FILL IN THE BLANK

Complete each statement by providing the word(s) missing where the blank is shown.

1. Health care _____ allows the population greater access to services that will allow them to stay healthy, treat minor illness or injury, and assess risk factors for certain types of diseases for which certain populations may be more susceptible.

2. Much of what pharmacy technicians learn about pharmacy benefits management is gained _____ _____ _____ collaborating with patients and the insurance companies that administer their pharmacy benefits.

3. Pharmacy technicians need to know how insurance works, as well as the basic _____ and _____ of health and pharmacy benefits that exist.

4. Pharmacy technicians need to know the law and possess the ability to explain _____ _____ as they relate to both federal and state legislation.

5. _____ _____ _____ is typically a family or general practitioner who is qualified to attend to most areas of preventive care and general wellness and to treat minor to moderate conditions.

6. Pharmacy technicians should verify prescription co-pay or co-insurance amounts, which may then be communicated and _____ to the patient.

7. It is important for a pharmacy technician to verify whether a plan requires a _____ and whether it has been met.

8. Pharmacy technicians should seek out resources for staying current on the basic plan structures as well as benefit eligibility _____ that must be met for patients to use their benefits.

9. When a claim is sent electronically, or _____, the insurance company will return an electronic response.

10. Pharmacy technicians must become familiar with claim _____ codes, as well as strategies for correcting them, to communicate appropriately with pharmacy benefit providers.

MATCHING

Match each pharmacy benefits term with its corresponding definition.

1. _____ Sets forth the types of benefits that the plan may allow, based on the beneficiary's eligibility

2. _____ Rejection on the part of the drug benefit provider to cover a particular medication, based on plan limitations or drug coverage restrictions

3. _____ A category of drug information that indicates interactions among various drugs or classes of drugs that may result in serious complications if the drugs are taken during the same course of therapy

4. _____ The process of switching an existing prescription to another—usually less expensive—medicine that is chemically different (not a generic) but is used to treat the same clinical condition

5. _____ A trademarked commercial name given to a generic drug product, often protected by drug patent

6. _____ A drug that does not have a trademarked name and is the therapeutic equivalent of a brand name drug, although it has been manufactured at a much lower cost

7. _____ A prescription medication for which a beneficiary's prescription drug benefit pays at least part of the cost during the plan year

8. _____ Steps that should be taken by a Medicare Part D beneficiary to request a reevaluation of a decision made about prescription coverage

9. _____ A form of drug benefit coverage determination that requires a prescriber to obtain advance approval for a particular product before the patient will receive benefit coverage

10. _____ A list of which medicines a benefit plan covers and at what level of co-payment

a. Appeal process

b. Brand name drug

c. Contraindication

d. Coverage determination

e. Covered drug

f. Denial

g. Formulary

h. Generic drug

i. Prior authorization

j. Therapeutic substitution

MULTIPLE CHOICE

Select the best answer for each question.

1. Which of the following is an example of a preexisting condition?
   a. Diabetes
   b. Cancer
   c. Asthma
   d. All of the above

2. _____ is a federal and state-sponsored insurance coverage plan for individuals with preexisting conditions who have been uninsured for at least 6 months.
   a. HMO
   b. PCIP
   c. PCP
   d. PPO

3. Medicare Part _____ covers preventive care as well as benefits for regular maintenance care in a physician's office. The plan covers provider services, hospital outpatient care, and home health care.
   a. A
   b. B
   c. C
   d. D

4. Medicare Part C Plans are also referred to as _____ and are provided by Medicare-approved private insurance companies.
   a. The "Donut-hole"
   b. Coverage Gap
   c. Medicare Advantage Plans
   d. Affordable Care

5. Benefit plans structured and managed by a pharmacy benefit management (PBM) company would include which of the following?
   a. WellPoint
   b. Express Scripts
   c. AdvancePCS
   d. All of the above

6. PBMs negotiate pricing based on several factors of key importance to their industry partners, including all of the following except _____.
   a. co-pay
   b. dispensing fees
   c. prior authorization
   d. therapeutic substitution

7. Specialty drugs, such as biologics or gene therapy, will typically be a Tier _____ drug on a tiered pricing structure.
   a. 1
   b. 2
   c. 3
   d. 4

8. PBMs usually partner with mail-order pharmacies to offer _____ day supply programs for maintenance drugs, as well as drugs for which patients are offered incentives for using the lower-cost generic versions.
   a. 30
   b. 60
   c. 90
   d. 120

9. When processing an electronic claim, the rejection code with the electronic adjudication response from the insurance company was "Date Written Is After Date Filled." What strategy would you use to resolve this?
   a. Verify information entered under the patient profile and update.
   b. Verify information entered in the pharmacy database.
   c. Verify provider eligibility with the benefit provider.
   d. Verify information entered under the prescriber profile.

10. When processing an electronic claim, the rejection code with the electronic adjudication response from the insurance company was "Invalid Date of Birth." What strategy would you use to resolve this?
    a. Verify information entered under the patient profile and update.
    b. Verify information entered in the pharmacy database.
    c. Verify provider eligibility with the benefit provider.
    d. Verify information entered under the prescriber profile.

CRITICAL THINKING

Based on what you have learned in the textbook, answer the following questions.

1. You receive a prescription for ibuprofen 600 mg, i po qid, dispense 84 tabs. When processing an electronic claim, the rejection code with the electronic adjudication response from the insurance company is "Days Supply Limitation for Product is 14 days." How would you resolve this rejection?

   _____

   _____

   _____

2. When processing an electronic claim the rejection code with the electronic adjudication response from the insurance company is "Prior Authorization Required." How could you help resolve this rejection?

   _____

   _____

   _____

INTERNET EXERCISES

Answer the following questions by researching your answers on the Internet.

1. Pharmacy technicians may need to conduct research with a PBM to determine a beneficiary's pricing for a particular medication. Research one of the PBMs listed in the chapter. How would knowing how to look up and determine a beneficiary's pricing for a particular medication be beneficial to your work practice?

_____

_____

_____

2. Pharmacy technicians need to stay current with their state Medicaid program. Research your state's Medicaid program. List at least two rules that your state Medicaid program has in place for pharmacy benefits.

_____

_____

_____

13 Cultural Competence: The Journey to Effective Communication in a Culturally Diverse Society

KEY TERMINOLOGY

Provide a definition for each term.

1. Active listening:

   _____

   _____

2. Bias:

   _____

   _____

3. Cultural imperialism:

   _____

   _____

4. Cultural norms:

   _____

   _____

5. Cultural relativism:

   _____

   _____

6. Culture:

   _____

   _____

7. Ethnic pluralism:

   _____

   _____

8. Ethnocentrism:

   _____

   _____

9. Media:

   _____

   _____

10. Message/feedback:

_____

_____

11. Message incongruence:

_____

_____

12. Prejudice:

_____

_____

13. Receiver:

_____

_____

14. Sender:

_____

_____

FILL IN THE BLANK

Complete each statement by providing the word(s) missing where the blank is shown.

1. It is important that pharmacy technicians recognize the factors that have influenced the formation of the patient's _____ or _____.

2. Message processing may be filtered by a person's _____ _____, which can strongly influence the receiver's response to the sender.

3. Because _____ _____ can be quite subjective, it is extremely important that the sender verify with the receiver that the message was received and interpreted as the sender intended.

4. In cases of message incongruence, it is important to ask a few simple, _____ _____ questions to help clarify what the person is truly trying to communicate.

5. Most people have experienced the frustration of attempting conversation with someone who was not actually _____ to them.

6. Active listening is crucial to _____ _____ in the health care setting.

7. Pharmacy technicians must _____, _____, and _____ their patterns of communication whenever necessary to suit the needs of a widely diverse patient population.

8. How people view their own _____ and _____ self may influence how they feel about and respond to individuals of other cultures.

9. An increased awareness of attitudes toward and perspectives on other cultures can make pharmacy technicians _____ _____ to how they treat patients who share their cultural backgrounds, in addition to those of different backgrounds.

10. Health care professionals, including pharmacy technicians, must find ways to acknowledge patients' _____ _____ of medicine when presenting patients with prescription medications.

MATCHING

Match each positive characteristic to practice when receiving feedback with its corresponding definition.

1. _____ Try to understand the personal behaviors and/or cultural norms that may influence the feedback.

2. _____ Accept the feedback without devaluing it.

3. _____ Show a genuine desire to make personal changes if they are appropriate.

4. _____ Interact with the speaker and ask for clarification when appropriate.

5. _____ Recognize the feedback's value and the value of the person who sent it.

a. Acceptance

b. Respect

c. Engagement

d. Thoughtfulness

e. Sincerity

Match each negative characteristic *not* to practice when receiving feedback with its corresponding definition.

6. _____ Listening and agreeing without intending to use the feedback to make any changes.

7. _____ Refuting the accuracy or fairness of the feedback.

8. _____ Finding explanations that remove personal responsibility.

9. _____ Defending one's personal actions and objecting to the feedback.

10. _____ Devaluing the speaker and the feedback provided.

a. Defensiveness

b. Denial

c. Disrespect

d. Rationalizing

e. Patronizing

MULTIPLE CHOICE

Select the best answer for each question.

1. _____ are usually based on outside individuals' perceptions and opinions, rather than on the viewpoint of the group.
   a. Cultural norms
   b. Biases
   c. Stereotypes
   d. Cultures

2. Which of the following would be an example of direct communication?
   a. Talking on the telephone
   b. Texting on a cell phone
   c. Sending a message by email
   d. All of the above

3. Which of the following would be an example of indirect communication?
   a. Rolling your eyes
   b. Sending a fax message
   c. Posting a memo on the bulletin board
   d. All of the above

4. When the sender's direct and indirect message is transmitted with a very different meaning from the perspective of the receiver, it is called _____.
   a. active listening
   b. incongruence
   c. closed-mindedness
   d. patronizing

5. As a pharmacy technician, which of the following behaviors can help you make sure you are actively listening?
   a. Allow the speaker to communicate without interruption.
   b. Establish appropriate eye contact.
   c. Provide the communicator with an outward indicator of your attention, such as a nod or other facial or nonverbal cue.
   d. All of the above

6. Which of the following is not a key element to cultural competence?
   a. Arrogance
   b. Attitude
   c. Skills of interpreting and relating
   d. Skills of discovery and interaction

7. External influences, often referred to as _____, may alter people's behavior in a way that may conflict with their own attitudes and beliefs, to please the majority or preserve the status quo.
   a. religion
   b. peer pressure
   c. life experiences
   d. culture misconceptions

8. One of the best ways to diffuse a misconception in a culturally diverse environment is to _____.
   a. gain knowledge to increase your awareness
   b. clarify it with facts
   c. improve your ability to interact more effectively
   d. All of the above

9. When communicating with a patient, you should _____.
   a. speak in technical language
   b. dominate the conversation
   c. gather as much pertinent information as possible to prevent patients from having to repeat themselves
   d. interrupt them when you know what they are trying to say

10. _____ can influence how we interpret information received.
    a. Cultural contexts
    b. Personal ideals
    c. Life experiences
    d. All of the above

CRITICAL THINKING

Based on what you have learned in the textbook, answer the following questions.

1. How does being aware of your own culture correlate with better communication in the pharmacy?

_____

_____

_____

2. How could you increase your own understanding and appreciation of other cultures?

_____

_____

_____

INTERNET EXERCISES

Answer the following questions by researching your answers on the Internet.

1. If a patient speaks English as a second language, it is best to use the services of a professional interpreter or another health care team member who speaks the same language as the patient. Research other resources online that could be utilized if an interpreter is not available.

_____

_____

_____

2. The Myers-Briggs assessment and the Jung Typology assessment are two examples mentioned in the chapter to determine personality typology. Search online for a personality test and fill out the questionnaire to help determine your personality typology. Using the results, research information on your types and other types. How can this information help you better communicate with others?

_____

_____

_____

14 Infection Control

KEY TERMINOLOGY

Provide a definition for each term.

1. Infection:

   _____

   _____

2. Infection reservoir:

   _____

   _____

3. Mode of transmission:

   _____

   _____

4. Nonpathogenic:

   _____

   _____

5. Nosocomial infection:

   _____

   _____

6. Pathogenic:

   _____

   _____

7. Personal protective equipment (PPE):

   _____

   _____

8. Susceptible host:

   _____

   _____

FILL IN THE BLANK

Complete each statement by providing the word(s) missing where the blank is shown.

1. Because the health care environment is constantly exposed to disease-causing agents, controlling the spread of infection is a matter of _____ _____.

2. Primary goals of the pharmacist and pharmacy technician practice that are related to infection control are the _____, _____, and _____ of pharmaceutical products that may be safely administered to and by patients.

3. The term _____ _____ implies that there will always be the possibility of infection—we must simply find ways to *control* the amount of infection and the extent to which it spreads.

4. It is critical for pharmacy technicians to be knowledgeable about how infection is spread and the behaviors that must be adopted to _____ that risk.

5. Based on epidemiological studies, a distance of approximately _____ _____ in diameter around an infected host would allow for direct droplet contact transmission of a respiratory bacterial or viral agent.

6. The type of reservoir in which the infecting agent has been transported often determines the _____ _____ _____.

7. Based on the transmission entry point, members of the health care team can employ measures to create _____ _____ that will safeguard both them and patients against transmission of disease through various portals of entry.

8. One of the most effective methods for preventing the spread of infection is proper _____ _____.

9. One of the best ways to avoid exposure to infectious disease when transmission-based precautions are in place is to _____ exposure to susceptible areas.

10. When the risk of serious infectious disease is present, pharmacy technicians should avoid contact with the affected areas unless their presence is _____ _____ to deliver essential care to the patient or service to a member of the nursing staff.

MATCHING

Match each disease with its corresponding mode of transmission.

1. _____ SARS

2. _____ Measles

3. _____ Malaria

4. _____ Flu

5. _____ Herpes

6. _____ Whooping cough

7. _____ Tuberculosis

8. _____ Strep respiratory infection

a. Direct or indirect contact

b. Droplet contact

c. Airborne

d. Vector-borne

MULTIPLE CHOICE

Select the best answer for each question.

1. _____ and _____ have established standards and guidelines that detail measures that may prevent infections associated with air, water, and other elements in the health care environment.
   a. OSHA and FDA
   b. FDA and CDC
   c. CDC and OSHA
   d. FDA and ACPE

2. Today's infectious disease control measures have been impacted by the emergence of particularly virulent pathogens, including _____.
   a. severe acute respiratory syndrome (SARS)
   b. swine flu
   c. methicillin-resistant *Staphylococcus aureus* (MRSA)
   d. All of the above

3. The term _____ refers to infections acquired in a setting other than the hospital.
   a. nosocomial infection
   b. health care–associated infection
   c. portal of entry
   d. contact transmission

4. How infection begins and is spread is commonly referred to as the _____.
   a. chain of infection
   b. nosocomial infection
   c. mode of transmission
   d. vector-borne transmission

5. _____ is the most common form of pathogen transmission.
   a. Vector-borne transmission
   b. Vehicle transmission
   c. Airborne transmission
   d. Contact transmission

6. Entry of blood or blood-containing fluids into the host's body after contact with the infected human reservoir source is an example of _____ transmission.
   a. direct
   b. indirect
   c. vector-borne
   d. airborne

7. Introduction of microbial or particulate contamination because of poor aseptic technique during the process of intravenous (IV) admixture is an example of _____ transmission.
   a. direct
   b. indirect
   c. vector-borne
   d. airborne

8. An infection contracted through an arthropod such as a tick, mosquito, or flea is an example of _____ transmission.
   a. direct
   b. indirect
   c. vector-borne
   d. airborne

9. When properly performed, the process of aseptic hand washing should take no more than _____ from start to finish.
   a. 30 seconds
   b. 1 minute
   c. 90 seconds
   d. 2 minutes

10. _____ are behaviors that all health care workers should observe to prevent the introduction and spread of contaminants among health care workers, patients, and the health care environment.
    a. Standard precautions
    b. Safety culture
    c. Aseptic technique
    d. Survival factors

CRITICAL THINKING

Based on what you have learned in the textbook, answer the following questions.

1. Standard precautions are behaviors that all health care workers should observe to prevent the introduction and spread of contaminants among health care workers, patients, and the health care environment. Unfortunately, the standard precautions may not always be followed properly each time. Explain the importance of standard precautions and why they should be followed at all times, no matter the circumstance.

   _____

   _____

   _____

2. Proper hygienic hand washing before and after contact with an area for which there is a transmission-based precaution is one of the best ways to minimize the risk of spreading the infection to other health care workers, patients, and other environments in the health care setting. Even though many health care workers know this to be true, many reasons have been given for poor adherence to proper hand-washing techniques. What methods could you use in daily practice to always perform proper hygienic hand washing when necessary?

   _____

   _____

   _____

INTERNET EXERCISES

Answer the following questions by researching your answers on the Internet.

1. Research standards and guidelines that detail measures specific to the practice of pharmacy established by the Occupational Safety and Health Administration (OSHA). What additional standards and guidelines are established for pharmacy practice?

   _____

   _____

   _____

2. Research the product GloGerm. How can this product be useful for infection control?

   _____

   _____

   _____

15 Pharmacy Materials Management

KEY TERMINOLOGY

Provide a definition for each term.

1. Acquisition cost:

_____

_____

2. Basic stock:

_____

_____

3. Carrying costs:

_____

_____

4. Discontinued:

_____

_____

5. Expired product:

_____

_____

6. Order cycle time:

_____

_____

7. Perpetual inventory management:

_____

_____

8. Procurement:

_____

_____

9. Procurement costs:

_____

_____

10. Purchase order:

_____

_____

11. Recalled product:

_____

_____

12. Safety stock:

_____

_____

FILL IN THE BLANK

Complete each statement by providing the word(s) missing where the blank is shown.

1. Whether in the community or hospital pharmacy setting, _____ _____ processes impact a pharmacy's ability to provide needed products and services to patients.

2. Key opportunities for advancement to the position of _____ _____ exist in both community and hospital pharmacy settings.

3. Managing prescription benefit _____ helps keep the overall costs for those services affordable for most patients.

4. Many pharmacy inventory management systems provide a formulary listing of products that the pharmacy stocks; products are generally listed by their _____ _____ _____.

5. Pharmacy shipments must never be placed on _____ _____ until all products have been properly received.

6. Vaccinations are an example of a range of products for which _____ _____ may be maintained.

7. Proper management of pharmacy inventory is critical for delivering patient care and optimizing a pharmacy's greatest asset: its _____ _____.

8. Deviations in the (drug) counts are counted as _____.

9. Short-dated items should be rotated to the _____ to ensure that they are dispensed first.

10. _____ _____ _____ allow for better tracking of inventory and permit more accurate product selection during the prescription order and fill process.

MATCHING

Match each pharmacy inventory storage temperature with its corresponding description.

1. _____ 46°F to 59°F

2. _____ 86°F to 104°F

3. _____ 36°F to 46°F

4. _____ More than 104°F

5. _____ 59°F to 86°F

a. Cold

b. Cool

c. Room temperature

d. Warm

e. Excessively hot

MULTIPLE CHOICE

Select the best answer for each question.

1. The pharmacy procurement process is a primary way to carrying out the _____ principle of the Code of Ethics for Pharmacy Technicians.
   a. first
   b. third
   c. eighth
   d. ninth

2. Which of the following is a key component of the pharmacy materials management process?
   a. Formulary selection
   b. Managing inventory
   c. Product recalls
   d. All of the above

3. Formularies are generally established by a(n) _____ that has been created within a community or hospital pharmacy organization.
   a. FDA
   b. P&T committee
   c. manufacturer
   d. inventory committee

4. A purchase from a _____ is generally the most costly option for pharmacies and is typically done only in emergency situations when a product is unavailable through any other approved source.
   a. drug manufacturer
   b. prime vendor
   c. wholesaler
   d. GPO

5. Same-day ordering may be accomplished through a _____, as long as the order is generated and transmitted by an established cutoff time.
   a. wholesaler
   b. GPO
   c. prime vendor
   d. drug manufacturer

6. Drug products account for _____ of the total budget allocation, thus making them the single greatest investment for a pharmacy organization.
   a. 50% to 60%
   b. 60% to 70%
   c. 70% to 80%
   d. 80% to 90%

7. Drug product loss may result from _____.
   a. product receiving errors
   b. restocking errors
   c. product damage
   d. All of the above

8. Cycle counting also allows pharmacy staff to verify that products are of the highest level of quality possible; this helps uphold the _____ principle of the Code of Ethics for Pharmacy Technicians.
   a. first
   b. third
   c. eighth
   d. ninth

9. _____ may request that a product be recalled, based on concerns about the product's efficacy, purity, or functionality.
   a. The FDA
   b. The drug manufacturer
   c. The product manufacturer
   d. All of the above

10. The most severe drug recall would be classified as a _____ because the product could lead to serious health consequences up to and including death.
    a. type 1
    b. type 2
    c. type 3
    d. type 4

CRITICAL THINKING

Based on what you have learned in the textbook, answer the following questions.

1. Using the following fee table, calculate the final dispensing price of a prescription for 30 tablets if a bottle of 100 tablets has an AWP of $48.65.

AWP	DISPENSING FEE
$0-$5.00	$2.75
$5.01-$10.00	$3.75
$10.01-$20.00	$4.75
$20.00 and up	$5.75

_____

_____

_____

2. You are the inventory pharmacy technician for your pharmacy. You are gathering information on two drug products to help the P&T committee decide which drug product would be the most cost effective. What is the pharmacy's cost savings per unit if lisinopril 20 mg is dispensed instead of quinapril 20 mg? Which product would you recommend as the most cost effective if the prices of both drugs from your supplier are as follows:

Lisinopril 20 mg tablets, 1000-count bottle: $1053.45

Quinapril 20 mg tablets, 500-count bottle: $785.40

_____

_____

_____

INTERNET EXERCISES

Answer the following questions by researching your answers on the Internet.

1. MedWatch is the FDA's safety information and adverse event report program. Go to the MedWatch website located at http://www.fda.gov/Safety/MedWatch/default.htm. Research latest recalls. Are there any type 1 recalls listed? What are the recommendations for resolving the recall?

_____

_____

_____

2. Research look-alike/sound-alike drug names. List at least five look-alike/sound-alike drug names you should be aware of when working in a pharmacy.

_____

_____

_____

16 Medication Safety and Error Prevention

KEY TERMINOLOGY

Provide a definition for each term.

1. Adverse drug event (ADE):

_____

_____

2. Medication error:

_____

_____

3. Medication misadventure:

_____

_____

FILL IN THE BLANK

Complete each statement by providing the word(s) missing where the blank is shown.

1. The _____ _____ of pharmacy technician practice is to support the pharmacist in the safe, efficacious dispensing of quality pharmaceutical products and services.

2. _____ _____ contribute to rising health care costs, and an alarming increase in the annual number of errors must be addressed aggressively, at every level of the medication order entry and fill process.

3. When an error occurs, pharmacy and other health care personnel have an _____ and a _____ obligation to report it.

4. Workflow must be managed properly to ensure that _____ is not compromised or abandoned in the pursuit of meeting workflow demands.

5. Pharmacy technicians must recognize that every task associated with pharmacy practice should be well documented as a process in the pharmacy's _____ _____ _____.

6. It is important to consider how medication errors may occur when observance of the five rights is _____.

7. Pharmacists and pharmacy technicians can help prevent medication errors and misadventures by learning from their _____.

8. The publication _____ _____ is designed for consumers and provides information on ways patients can help prevent medication errors and misadventures through communication with their caregivers and pharmacists and through sources of health care education.

9. _____ by the pharmacy often prevents lawsuits.

10. All individuals involved in the medication error should complete any necessary internal documentation and provide as much _____ as possible.

MATCHING

Match each patient right of medication administration with its corresponding medication error resulting from a breakdown in adherence.

1. _____ Wrong product with a similar name selected

2. _____ Wrong IV drip flow rate entered and noted on an IV solution label

3. _____ Wrong concentration strength of a liquid drug

4. _____ Wrong patient's refill number selected

5. _____ Incorrect otic or ophthalmic product selected

6. _____ Similar or multiple names in a database without distinguishing patient identifiers

7. _____ Wrong release rate of a product selected

8. _____ Intravenous (IV) administration of an oral drug

9. _____ Wrong form of the right drug selected

10. _____ Wrong administration interval entered on an IV solution label

a. Right patient

b. Right drug

c. Right dose

d. Right route

e. Right time

MULTIPLE CHOICE

Select the best answer for each question.

1. A medication misadventure caused by the pharmacy may be an event that _____.
   a. occurs when the medication is given incorrectly
   b. occurs when the medication is self-administered incorrectly
   c. harms a patient because of a fill error
   d. results from a prescription that was filled incorrectly

2. An example of an internal stressor that may lead to a medication error would include _____.
   a. customer traffic
   b. incoming telephone calls
   c. similar drug names
   d. no one available to double check

3. An example of an external stressor that may lead to a medication error would include _____.
   a. illegible prescriptions
   b. staff shortage
   c. lack of concentration
   d. no time to counsel

4. _____ would be an example of a communication breakdown that could lead to a medication error.
   a. Spelling and order entry errors resulting from lack of attention
   b. Incorrect transcription during a verbal order
   c. Use of visual product recognition instead of reading the label
   d. Difficult to read storage labeling

5. _____ would be an example of an inventory storage practice that could lead to a medication error.
   a. Shortcuts or poor techniques that develop over time
   b. Use of visual product recognition instead of reading the label
   c. Improper pass-down of information
   d. Incorrect product locations

6. _____ would be an example of a repetition or acquired blindness habit that could lead to a medication error.
   a. Spelling and order entry errors resulting from lack of attention
   b. Look-alike or sound-alike products stored close together
   c. Poor or inadequate lighting in drug storage areas
   d. Illegible handwriting that is not verified for clarification

7. The abbreviation _____ is often mistaken as "mg," which would result in an overdose.
   a. mcg
   b. μg
   c. g
   d. ɱg

8. The abbreviation _____ is often mistaken as "U" when poorly written.
   a. IU
   b. IV
   c. cc
   d. Q

9. _____ is a U.S. Food and Drug Administration (FDA) program to report serious ADEs.
   a. *FDA Drug Safety Newsletter*
   b. *Nurse Advise-ERR*
   c. Medication Errors Reporting Program (MERP)
   d. MedWatch Program

10. When an error occurs, the pharmacy files a detailed report with the _____, which is a part of the U.S. Pharmacopeia/Institute for Safe Medication Practices (USP-ISMP).
   a. MedWatch Program
   b. Medication Errors Reporting Program (MERP)
   c. *FDA Drug Safety Newsletter*
   d. *Safe Medicine* publication

CRITICAL THINKING

Based on what you have learned in the textbook, answer the following questions.

1. An order for famotidine 20 mg IV q12h (0800 and 2000) is written. The initial dose is administered at 1000. Which patient right has been compromised?

_____

_____

_____

2. An order is received for Paxil 40 mg po qam. The pharmacy dispenses paroxetine 40 mg tablets to the patient with a translated sig of: Take 1 tablet by mouth every evening. Which patient right has been compromised?

_____

_____

_____

INTERNET EXERCISES

Answer the following questions by researching your answers on the Internet.

1. Research medication misadventures on the ISMP website located at www.ismp.org. List at least two medication misadventures that can help you perform better while working as a pharmacy technician.

_____

_____

_____

2. Research Emily's Law. How can this very tragic medication misadventure help you be more diligent to protecting and adhering to the patient rights of medication administration?

_____

_____

_____

17 The Structure and Organization of Institutional Pharmacy Practice

KEY TERMINOLOGY

Provide a definition for each term.

1. Decentralized service:

   _____

   _____

2. Health system:

   _____

   _____

3. Medication reconciliation:

   _____

   _____

4. Triage:

   _____

   _____

FILL IN THE BLANK

Complete each statement by providing the word(s) missing where the blank is shown.

1. Individuals who provide pharmaceutical products in an institutional pharmacy not only serve patients, but also strongly affect the capability of _____ members of the health care team to serve patients.

2. A hospital may be considered an establishment that offers services to help maintain the health and vitality of a local community or _____ _____.

3. The hospital organization involves a variety of services that support patient care, employees, and the physical hospital environment to establish a _____ _____ _____.

4. The process of _____ _____ is an extremely important part of establishing a patient's medical history.

5. The _____ _____ is the main source of pharmaceutical products, services, and clinical support for the hospital.

6. The _____ _____, a national organization that accredits hospitals and health organizations, has established rules for preparing medications.

7. Patient care areas that serve a specific patient population or patients who need a narrow range of products and services may be provided by a decentralized _____ _____, which is a scaled-down version of the central pharmacy.

8. The Joint Commission site surveyors may inquire about a pharmacy staff member's knowledge of his or her facility's safety policy or procedures, so pharmacy technicians should stay _____.

9. In the central pharmacy, orders most often are transmitted _____ or by _____.

10. The use of _____ _____ helps to enhance the role of the hospital pharmacy in patient care because it allows pharmacists to spend more time providing consultation services to the health care teams in patient care areas.

MATCHING

Match each institutional pharmacy duty with a pharmacy technician's ability to perform or not perform it.

1. _____ Preparing drug carts or trays

2. _____ Answering and directing phone calls

3. _____ Aseptically mixing parenteral products

4. _____ Speaking to a nurse about a patient's medical condition and suggesting which medications should be discontinued

5. _____ Removing overstocks

6. _____ Delivering controlled drugs

7. _____ Recommending a dosage adjustment based on the patient's weight or condition

8. _____ Counting and pouring medication

9. _____ Advising a patient to continue taking a medication after discharge

10. _____ Weighing and measuring bulk materials

a. May perform

b. May *not* perform

MULTIPLE CHOICE

Select the best answer for each question.

1. The institutional pharmacy focuses primarily on _____.
   a. dispensing medication
   b. patient counseling
   c. scheduled distribution of pharmaceutical products
   d. All of the above

2. In an institutional pharmacy setting, _____ is one of the primary customers for pharmacy staff.
   a. the patient
   b. the nurse
   c. housekeeping
   d. the respiratory therapist

3. Medication orders to be reviewed and verified by a pharmacist in a hospital setting can be received by all of the following methods *except* _____.
   a. dropped off by a patient
   b. entered manually
   c. entered electronically
   d. transmitted by fax

4. Medications in a hospital setting are generally distributed to the following areas:
   a. Patient's bedside
   b. Restricted-access medication storage room
   c. Automated dispensing machine
   d. All of the above

5. Which of the following clinical areas in a hospital may have a satellite pharmacy?
   a. Radiology
   b. Speech pathology
   c. Oncology
   d. Dietary services

6. The Joint Commission established _____ to address areas of key concern in patient safety across health care systems.
   a. bloodborne pathogen tests
   b. National Patient Safety Goals
   c. OSHA standards
   d. aseptic technique standards

7. Hospital pharmacies may generally dispense a _____ supply of medication in a blister pack card to nursing home residents for medication support.
   a. 14- to 21-day
   b. 30-day
   c. 3-month
   d. 6-month

8. If an order is for a *STAT* medication, the drug must be administered within _____ or less from the time the order was written.
   a. 1 hour
   b. 45 minutes
   c. 30 minutes
   d. 1 minute

9. Pharmacy technicians who want to be considered for the job of checking technician must undergo extensive training that includes subjects such as _____.
   a. Medication therapy management
   b. Pharmacology
   c. Techniques for preventing medication errors
   d. All of the above

10. After a checking technician has completed training, he or she typically must demonstrate skill in checking filled medication doses by achieving an accuracy rate of _____ or better.
    a. 100%
    b. 99.7%
    c. 98%
    d. 95%

CRITICAL THINKING

Based on what you have learned in the textbook, answer the following questions.

1. Medication reconciliation is a fairly new career opportunity that has allowed some pharmacy technicians to move out of the pharmacy and into the emergency department. How could your knowledge as a pharmacy technician be beneficial in this new role? How could having prior community pharmacy practice be an asset to obtaining a position as a medication reconciliation technician?

   _____

   _____

   _____

2. A TJC surveyor (inspector) may visit an accredited facility at any time to verify that a hospital's organizational structure and processes are consistent with the established standards. For pharmacy technicians, it is important to be aware of key compliance issues, such as:

   ■ How frequently training is conducted

   ■ Instances in which a pharmacist needs to check his or her work

   ■ How often quality assurance processes (e.g., expiration date checks and cleaning) are conducted

   ■ How errors are handled, documented, and corrected

   How can you help your pharmacy be aware of these key compliance issues so that the pharmacy will always be prepared for an impromptu visit from a TJC inspector?

   _____

   _____

   _____

INTERNET EXERCISES

Answer the following questions by researching your answers on the Internet.

1. Various state boards of pharmacy may specifically define what constitutes institutional pharmacy practice in their state. Research your state to verify your state's specific definition of institutional practice.

_____

_____

_____

2. The use of pharmacy technicians as checking technicians is good for the profession because it does not require clinical decision making, which will improve a pharmacists' ability to serve patients and creates an excellent opportunity for career advancement for pharmacy technicians. Research your state's regulations on allowing the use of checking technicians. Is this an opportunity your state allows or is it something that is beginning to be discussed?

_____

_____

_____

18 Institutional Pharmacy Practice II: Drug Distribution Systems

KEY TERMINOLOGY

Provide a definition for each term.

1. Automation:

2. Drug distribution system:

3. Prepackage:

4. Repackage:

5. Unit dose:

6. Unit-dose cart fill:

FILL IN THE BLANK

Complete each statement by providing the word(s) missing where the blank is shown.

1. The outcome of hospital pharmacy workflow is drug _____.

2. The process in which patient-specific doses are prepared in individual packaging and distributed to patient-specific storage areas is called a unit-dose cart fill, or _____ _____ for short.

3. For _____ _____ _____, automation plays a critical role in patient-specific dose dispensing because doses are more readily available for administration by a patient caregiver.

4. Individual patient profiling improves _____ for each scheduled dose and reduces the number of doses dispensed incorrectly.

5. Once the pharmacist check has been performed, the verified doses can be _____ to patient care areas.

6. Unit-dose packaging preserves the physical and chemical _____ of the product.

7. Pharmacy technicians involved in drug packaging must _____ make sure that a pharmacist has verified each dose packaged before the drug is distributed to pharmacy drug storage areas or to medication storage in patient care areas.

8. Proper drug storage systems allow for better _____ _____ and ensure that drugs are kept under conditions that maintain their stability.

9. Access to automated dispensing machines must be _____ to pharmacy staff members and authorized individuals who have been trained and are directly involved in patient care and medication administration.

10. To ensure patients' safety, a _____ _____ label is generated and affixed to any patient-specific dose that originates in the pharmacy.

MATCHING

Match each drug dispensing system with its corresponding manufacturer.

1. _____ MDG Medical

2. _____ AmerisourceBergen

3. _____ Metro

4. _____ MTS

5. _____ McKesson

6. _____ Talyst

7. _____ Cardinal Health

a. AutoPharm

b. MedDispense

c. MedSelect

d. AcuDose

e. MTS MedLocker

f. Serve Rx

g. Pyxis MedStation 3500

MULTIPLE CHOICE

Select the best answer for each question.

1. Automation has improved which of the following key areas of pharmacy practice?
   a. Patient safety
   b. Inventory control
   c. Workflow efficiency
   d. All of the above

2. When implementing technology in the distribution of medications, _____ is expected to be the primary goal.
   a. convenience
   b. patient safety
   c. efficiency
   d. All of the above

3. Because prescribers' orders may change frequently, patients in a hospital are typically dispensed no more than a _____ hour supply.
   a. 6-
   b. 12-
   c. 24-
   d. 48-

4. The pharmacy technician's duties when working with a medication carousel include _____.
   a. stocking, checking expiration dates, and verifying product inventory counts
   b. picking doses for distribution
   c. checking doses if trained as a checking technician
   d. All of the above

5. Robotic systems can streamline a large batch fill and can reduce 3- to 4-hour medication pick and fill processes to approximately _____, thereby decreasing the turnaround time for delivery to the patients.
   a. 45 minutes
   b. 90 minutes
   c. 120 minutes
   d. 150 minutes

6. Medication can be removed from an automated dispensing machine by _____.
   a. patient name
   b. individual product
   c. room number
   d. a and c

7. Hospital regulatory standards require that doses be verified by a _____ before dispensing.
   a. nurse
   b. physician
   c. pharmacist
   d. pharmacy technician

8. Hospital pharmacy and therapeutics (P&T) committees generally establish a list of drugs used in acute care or that may be appropriate in emergencies; these drugs are commonly referred to as _____.
   a. exception drugs
   b. override drugs
   c. exclusion drugs
   d. omission drugs

9. At least _____, pharmacists and pharmacy technicians must inventory all the drug pockets and drawers of each dispensing machine.
   a. monthly
   b. quarterly
   c. biannually
   d. yearly

10. When verifying inventory of all the drug pockets and drawers of each dispensing machine, you should also inspect the content to verify _____.
    a. placement of products in their correct location
    b. product expiration dates
    c. product packaging to ensure it has not been compromised or damaged
    d. All of the above

CRITICAL THINKING

Based on what you have learned in the textbook, answer the following questions.

1. Explain the importance of accounting for each unit-dose packaged medication.

   _____

   _____

   _____

2. As you have read in the chapter, automated machines are not only able to package solid unit doses such as tablets and capsules, but they can also package liquid unit doses into syringes. With this technology available to pharmacies, do you think pharmacy technicians may still be needed in a hospital setting?

   _____

   _____

   _____

INTERNET EXERCISES

Answer the following questions by researching your answers on the Internet.

1. Each state's board of pharmacy establishes standards of practice for the use of technology in pharmacy processes. Research your state's standard of practice for the use of technology in pharmacy processes. What types of technology is your state allowing?

   _____

   _____

   _____

2. Various drug dispensing systems are currently available, and many more are likely to reach the market as this technology continues to advance. Research one of the drug dispensing systems listed in the chapter. What specific features could help improve continuity of care?

   _____

   _____

   _____

19 Aseptic Admixture and Compounding Sterile Preparations

KEY TERMINOLOGY

Provide a definition for each term.

1. Ante-area:

   _____

   _____

2. Aseptic admixture:

   _____

   _____

3. Aseptic hand washing:

   _____

   _____

4. Aspirate:

   _____

   _____

5. Bactericidal:

   _____

   _____

6. Bacteriostatic:

   _____

   _____

7. Barrel:

   _____

   _____

8. Bevel:

   _____

   _____

9. Buffer area:

   _____

   _____

10. Chemical stability:

   _____

   _____

11. Controlled environment:

   _____

   _____

12. Gauge:

   _____

   _____

13. Heel:

   _____

   _____

14. HEPA filter:

   _____

   _____

15. Hub:

   _____

   _____

16. Hypertonicity:

   _____

   _____

17. Hypotonicity:

   _____

   _____

18. Isotonicity:

   _____

   _____

19. IV admixture:

   _____

   _____

20. Lumen:

   _____

   _____

21. Microbiologic stability:

_____

_____

22. Multiple-dose container:

_____

_____

23. Needles:

_____

_____

24. Open system:

_____

_____

25. Pass-throughs:

_____

_____

26. Pharmacy engineering control (PEC) devices:

_____

_____

27. Physical stability:

_____

_____

28. Plunger:

_____

_____

29. Quality assurance (QA):

_____

_____

30. Quality control (QC):

_____

_____

31. Response time:

_____

_____

32. Single-dose container:

_____

_____

33. Sterile:

_____

_____

34. Syringe:

_____

_____

35. Therapeutic stability:

_____

_____

36. Toxicologic stability:

_____

_____

FILL IN THE BLANK

Complete each statement by providing the word(s) missing where the blank is shown.

1. For a pharmacy technician, the ability to perform _____ _____ of sterile intravenous products is one of the most sought after and marketable hands-on skills.

2. The best way to protect patients is to minimize the chances of _____ _____ _____, which occur as a result of contamination of medication prepared by pharmacy staff members.

3. The purpose of compounding standards is to prevent the introduction and spread of contaminants into _____ _____ _____.

4. PPE for aseptic admixture is also commonly referred to as _____ _____ _____ and _____.

5. The laminar airflow workbench (LAFW) is commonly referred to as the _____ _____.

6. Aseptic compounding must take place 3 to 6 inches from the outer edge of the IV hood on the work surface, or what is known as the _____ _____.

7. A _____ _____ allows free transfer of a sterile solution into a syringe.

8. Cleansing of all surfaces within the clean room and ante-areas should be done _____.

9. You should perform air sampling of doorways or areas with significant air turbulence or that present opportunities for contamination every _____ _____.

10. The standard isotonic solution of sodium chloride is 0.9%, which is also known as _____ _____.

MATCHING

Match each step of donning personal protective equipment (PPE) with its correct procedural order.

1. _____ Put on head and facial hair covers.

2. _____ Put on nonshedding gown.

3. _____ Put on face masks and eye shields.

4. _____ Put on dedicated shoes or shoe covers.

5. _____ Put on sterile, powder-free gloves.

6. _____ Perform hand-cleansing procedures.

a. Step 1

b. Step 2

c. Step 3

d. Step 4

e. Step 5

f. Step 6

MULTIPLE CHOICE

Select the best answer for each question.

1. The first legally enforceable standard for sterile products that applied across the profession of pharmacy and was established by the USP is _____.
   a. USP Chapter <795>
   b. USP Chapter <797>
   c. USP Chapter <71>
   d. USP Chapter <621>

2. The space in which sterile medications are prepared may be referred to as a(n) _____.
   a. IV room
   b. controlled environment
   c. clean room
   d. All of the above

3. The _____ is where label preparation takes place, as well as hand washing and garbing.
   a. buffer area
   b. controlled environment
   c. ante-area
   d. pass-throughs

4. The _____ is where the sterile pharmaceuticals are actually prepared and must be maintained under ISO Class 7 conditions at all times.
   a. buffer area
   b. controlled environment
   c. ante-area
   d. pass-throughs

5. The HEPA filter, which removes particulates but not vapors or gases, must be checked every _____.
   a. month
   b. 3 months
   c. 6 months
   d. year

6. To create ISO Class 5 air quality, the LAFW must run continuously for at least _____ before use.
   a. 15 minutes
   b. 30 minutes
   c. 1 hour
   d. 2 hours

7. CSPs considered medium risk involve more opportunities for the introduction of contaminants or additional time for the growth of bacteria and should therefore be stored at room temperature no longer than _____.
   a. 45 days
   b. 9 days
   c. 48 hours
   d. 30 hours

8. A filter needle must be no larger than _____ to prevent the transfer of particulate matter.
   a. 5 microns
   b. 0.1 micron
   c. 0.2 micron
   d. 0.22 micron

9. Which of the following would be an effective antimicrobial solution for aseptic hand washing?
   a. 70% isopropyl alcohol
   b. 10% povidone-iodine
   c. Chlorhexidine gluconate
   d. All of the above

10. When cleaning the horizontal laminar, you should clean the sides of the hood in a _____ motion.
    a. circular
    b. horizontal
    c. vertical
    d. unmethodical

CRITICAL THINKING

Based on what you have learned in the textbook, answer the following questions.

1. The emergency room nurse has called the pharmacy to ask what the BUD should be for the IV bag she made for a patient for immediate use. She tells you the IV rate is 100 mL/hour for 4 hours. What BUD date should you tell the nurse to place on the IV bag?

   _____

   _____

   _____

2. A medication order is received in the pharmacy for vancomycin 500 mg IV q12h. You have a 1-g vial of vancomycin and have reconstituted it to a concentration of 100 mg/mL for IV administration. How many milliliters of vancomycin will you draw up to prepare the IV bag?

   _____

   _____

   _____

INTERNET EXERCISES

Answer the following questions by researching your answers on the Internet.

1. Research job opportunities in your area for IV admixture pharmacy technicians. What type of training and skills are pharmacy employers requiring pharmacy technicians to possess for this type of position?

   _____

   _____

   _____

2. Research IV admixture and sterile compounding requirements for your state. Does your state require IV admixture and sterile compounding certification to prepare sterile compounds? If so, what are the requirements to obtain IV admixture and sterile compounding certification?

   _____

   _____

   _____

20 Green Pharmacy Practice

KEY TERMINOLOGY

Provide a definition for each term.

1. Green pharmacy practice:

_____

_____

2. Sustainable health care culture:

_____

_____

FILL IN THE BLANK

Complete each statement by providing the word(s) missing where the blank is shown.

1. Among the key goals of many health care organizations is the implementation of processes that optimize patient care while _____ _____.

2. Specifically, green pharmacy practice focuses on the utilization of resources that allow for the proper handling and processing of _____ _____.

3. Pharmacy technicians can contribute to green pharmacy practice by demonstrating environmentally conscious _____ processes that reduce pharmaceutical waste pollution and conserve energy.

4. Pharmacy technicians should remind patients _____ to flush unused medication in the toilet.

5. The profession of pharmacy may further advance its organizations' sustainability by partnering with vendors that utilize _____ _____ processes.

6. A _____ _____ would perform a baseline assessment of a pharmacy organization's operations to identify potential cost savings, recommend green practices that could be reasonably implemented across the organization, and provide recommendations on how that organization can obtain certification through a third party.

7. _____ _____ is one measure that may reduce the overall carbon footprint of an organization.

8. The _____ impact of pharmaceutical care continues to be monitored and measured as innovation progresses.

9. The agricultural and livestock industries inadvertently contribute PIE through the practice of injecting _____ to increase livestock production.

10. Prescription take-back programs may be implemented on a larger scale to encourage consumers to practice safe disposal of unused and expired pharmaceuticals on a _____ basis.

MATCHING

Match each organization with its corresponding acronym.

1. _____ Drug Enforcement Agency
2. _____ U.S. Department of Agriculture
3. _____ Food and Drug Administration
4. _____ U.S. Fish and Wildlife Service
5. _____ Environmental Protection Agency

a. FDA
b. EPA
c. DEA
d. USDA
e. USFS

MULTIPLE CHOICE

Select the best answer for each question.

1. The _____ has set forth a variety of guidelines pertaining to the disposal of both hazardous and nonhazardous waste materials in the health care environment.
   a. USP
   b. FDA
   c. EPA
   d. ISMP

2. The improper disposal of expired or unused medication remains an ongoing consumer issue, sometimes referred to as PIE, or _____.
   a. prescriptions in the ecosystem
   b. pharmaceuticals in the environment
   c. prescriptions in the environment
   d. pharmaceuticals in the ecosystem

3. Green pharmacy practice in a community setting is measured by the ability of both independent and corporate pharmacy organizations to _____.
   a. reduce pharmaceutical waste
   b. educate consumers on the importance of proper disposal of medications
   c. provide consumers with a solution by setting up medication take-back programs
   d. All of the above

4. Green pharmacy practice in a hospital setting is measured by the ability of the department of pharmacy to become a more sustainable operation through education and training of green pharmacy practices such as _____.
   a. purchasing of more green products
   b. setting up recycling programs for glass, plastic, and paper products
   c. ordering supplies from manufacturers that provide these types of products and are geared more toward sustainability
   d. All of the above

5. Community pharmacies may obtain green certification through certifying agencies such as _____.
   a. Eco-Path Texas
   b. Leadership in Energy and Environmental Design (LEED)
   c. Green Globe
   d. All of the above

6. A green pharmacy certification focuses primarily on the reduction of pharmaceutical waste through _____.
   a. measuring the quantity of prescriptions filled
   b. medication take-back programs
   c. patient education
   d. All of the above

7. Reduction of unnecessary printing or double-sided printing can help save _____.
   a. paper
   b. energy
   c. time
   d. a and c

8. _____ are believed to be a large contributor to pharmaceutical metabolite waste entering the sewer system.
   a. Residential neighborhoods
   b. Local schools
   c. Family pets
   d. Drug manufacturing companies

9. According to the *Newsweek* 2010 rankings of U.S. companies, _____ was the leading company in green manufacturing practices.
   a. Pfizer
   b. Johnson & Johnson
   c. Eli Lilly
   d. Abbott Laboratories

10. The _____ industry plays a huge role in seeking opportunities to reduce pollution and groundwater contamination that occurs as a result of human sewage products.
    a. livestock
    b. farming
    c. drug manufacturing
    d. All of the above

CRITICAL THINKING

Based on what you have learned in the textbook, answer the following questions.

1. As a pharmacy technician, what role can you play in helping seek solutions to the impact of pharmaceuticals in the environment (PIE)?

_____

_____

_____

2. Your pharmacy will be sponsoring a medication take-back day and has designated you as official promoter. Design a sign or brochure or talking points about the event to help educate patients and to get them involved.

_____

_____

_____

INTERNET EXERCISES

Answer the following questions by researching your answers on the Internet.

1. Research the guidelines the FDA has helped establish for drug disposal. What are a few suggestions the FDA offers to help with the disposal of unused or expired medications?

_____

_____

_____

2. Research the National Prescription Drug Take-Back Day. When has the DEA scheduled the next national take-back day?

_____

_____

_____

21 Preparing for What Lies Ahead: The Technician Career Path Overview

KEY TERMINOLOGY

Provide a definition for each term.

1. Radiopharmaceuticals:

   _____

   _____

2. Telepharmacy:

   _____

   _____

FILL IN THE BLANK

Complete each statement by providing the word(s) missing where the blank is shown.

1. Those who began their practice with _____ _____ are postured to be the most competitive, given projected changes to the pharmacy technician practice.

2. The role of the pharmacist continues to evolve, thus creating more opportunities for the _____ of the pharmacy technician career path.

3. The rural hospital practice setting is one area with wide applications for electronic monitoring because of the overwhelming need for _____ _____.

4. The _____ need for a remote monitoring system is to allow a hospital or health system with a critical pharmacist staffing issue to provide patient care and safety.

5. _____ contain radioactive isotopes that help to identify the presence of disease in the human body and to diagnose diseases that affect every major human body system, including organs, vessels, and cellular structures.

6. Individuals who wish to pursue a career in _____ _____ may begin by seeking out opportunities to become involved in the orientation and training of new employees in their practice setting.

7. The first step to selling yourself is to write an appealing advertisement, or _____, that will convince an employer to want to buy what you're selling.

8. Résumé _____ should be brief, specific, and powerful.

9. Ensure, when job seeking, that you keep with you information needed to complete an application, such as job history information and _____ information.

10. Strive to present yourself as open, _____, and _____.

MATCHING

Match the interview styles with their corresponding descriptions.

1. _____ May include touring a facility and speaking with individuals who may be involved in the hiring decision or with whom you may work and on whom it would be useful to make a good impression

2. _____ An interview based on answers from past behavior to predict future behavior or performance

3. _____ Meeting with multiple individuals who are likely involved in the hiring decision

4. _____ A process of prescreening qualified applicants to help determine candidates for a live interview

a. Board/panel interview

b. Onsite interview

c. Behavioral interview

d. Telephone interview

MULTIPLE CHOICE

Select the best answer for each question.

1. Employment of pharmacy technicians is projected to increase by _____, and that will only increase as qualified, well-trained pharmacy technicians elevate their careers to more innovative and specialized roles in the health care and pharmacy practice settings.
   a. 20%
   b. 25%
   c. 31%
   d. 51%

2. As of July 2010, which of the following states have regulations in place related to telepharmacy?
   a. Texas
   b. North Dakota
   c. Idaho
   d. All of the above

3. One of the pharmacy technician's roles in the PBM setting is to _____.
   a. offer clinical consultative support and drug therapy analysis
   b. assist members with benefits claims processing
   c. design individual drug benefit plans
   d. negotiate contract relationships between community pharmacies and PBM organizations

4. Key knowledge-based competencies for nuclear pharmacy technicians include an understanding of _____.
   a. procedures and operations related to the reconstitution, packaging, and labeling of radiopharmaceuticals
   b. usual technician functions associated with a specific radiopharmacy entity
   c. manipulative and record-keeping functions associated with the compounding and dispensing of radiopharmaceuticals
   d. All of the above

5. A career opportunity for pharmacy technicians who possess a 4-year undergraduate degree may be available in the area of _____.
   a. pharmaceutical sales
   b. nuclear pharmacy
   c. telepharmacy
   d. None of the above

6. The _____ is currently the only professional organization that accredits pharmacy technician training programs.
   a. PTCB
   b. NABP
   c. ASHP
   d. NPTA

7. A basic résumé should include the following elements *except* _____.
   a. a contact phone number
   b. an e-mail address that will not leave a positive impression
   c. experience that is relevant to the position for which you are applying
   d. educational background in reverse chronological order

8. Proofread your résumé to ensure _____.
   a. there are no grammatical, punctuation, or typographical errors
   b. font type and size are consistent
   c. all action verb tenses are consistent
   d. All of the above

9. You do not have to wait for a personal invitation to interview or follow up on a submitted application because it is acceptable to follow up _____ if you have not heard anything to ask how long one should reasonably wait before following up.
   a. a few days later after the interview
   b. 1 day after the interview
   c. 1 hour after the interview
   d. the evening of the interview

10. Which of the following should you do before an interview?
    a. Practice speaking slowly and clearly.
    b. Practice good posture and a seated position that you will find comfortable during the interview.
    c. Sit in front of a mirror and rehearse sample interview responses.
    d. All of the above

CRITICAL THINKING

Based on what you have learned in the textbook, answer the following questions.

1. Which of the following innovative roles for pharmacy technicians listed in Box 21-2 most interests you? What type of additional training do you think you may need? How would this role contribute to the changing role of pharmacy as a health care provider?

   _____

   _____

   _____

2. Using the information presented about résumés, put your résumé together. What information would you highlight about yourself?

   _____

   _____

   _____

INTERNET EXERCISES

Answer the following questions by researching your answers on the Internet.

1. Research pharmacy jobs in your area. If you are ready, use the résumé you created from the previous section to begin applying for the job opportunities you found and are interested in.

   _____

   _____

   _____

2. Research telepharmacy and nuclear pharmacies in your area. Are there any in your area? If so, is this a pharmacy setting you would be interested in working in?

   _____

   _____

   _____

22 Identifying Quality Leadership and CQI Process Management in Pharmacy Practice

KEY TERMINOLOGY

Provide a definition for each term.

1. Leadership:

   _____

   _____

2. Management:

   _____

   _____

FILL IN THE BLANK

Complete each statement by providing the word(s) missing where the blank is shown.

1. Quality patient care _____ the benefits that patients gain from their medical and pharmaceutical treatment.

2. Pharmacy technicians are beginning to take on some of the _____ aspects of the pharmacy practice and are playing an increasingly important role in the delivery of pharmacy services.

3. The expanding role of the pharmacy technician includes _____, whether leading a practice, leading a shift, or leading a project.

4. The advancement of the pharmacy technician career path must be leveraged with higher quality standards in light of the increased industry demands for _____ patient care.

5. Although a leader may determine what an organization wishes to accomplish, a manager determines _____ the organization, and its employees will accomplish its mission.

6. Of the many requirements and expectations of the customer, pharmacists and pharmacy technicians must ensure that patient safety is always the _____ priority.

7. Pharmacy technicians must be aware of the causes of _____ _____ as well as the ways to prevent them and reduce the risk that errors will occur.

8. Medication errors are caused by system or process flaws and conditions that lead people to make mistakes or fail to _____ them.

9. Pharmacy technicians should take pride and personal _____ for the quality of the product or service they deliver.

10. When a medication error occurs, it is important to reflect on the causes of the error and _____ processes so that subsequent errors can be prevented.

MATCHING

Match each factor that may contribute to system failures in the medication use process with its corresponding example.

1. _____ Reconstituting a powdered drug with an incorrect amount of diluent

2. _____ Translating qid as qd when filling a prescription

3. _____ Filling a medication order without prescriber approval

4. _____ Refilling a prescription that does not have any refills

5. _____ Receiving a medication order that is illegible

6. _____ Measuring an IV medication dose incorrectly when compounding an IV bag

7. _____ Giving a prescription order to the incorrect patient when the patient is picking it up at the pharmacy

8. _____ Receiving a prescription for a drug strength that is unavailable

9. _____ Distributing expired medications to patients

10. _____ Administering a medication dose that is greater than the prescribed dose

a. Prescribing

b. Transcribing/documentation

c. Dispensing

d. Administration

MULTIPLE CHOICE

Select the best answer for each question.

1. Characteristics of a good leader include _____.
   a. the ability to help others see the immediate need for change
   b. the ability to understand the consequences of not acting or moving toward needed change
   c. the ability to convince others not to stand still and to move out of their comfort zone
   d. All of the above

2. Those chosen to be on the guiding team of a change management process should be able to _____.
   a. communicate effectively
   b. motivate others
   c. not be shy
   d. All of the above

3. A pharmacy manager's consistent oversight of the pharmacy technician's not using the new drug order log book demonstrates this step in the change management process:
   a. Enabling action
   b. Hold gains
   c. Short-term wins
   d. Coalition

4. A pharmacy manager's insistence that all pharmacy technicians ask an open-ended question to verify customer identity every time a customer picks up a prescription demonstrates this step in the change management process:
   a. Coalition
   b. Hold gains
   c. Short-term wins
   d. Anchor culture

5. By leading quality and safety in your pharmacy, you are upholding the _____ principle of the Code of Ethics for Pharmacy Technicians.
   a. third
   b. fifth
   c. eighth
   d. tenth

6. The ultimate goal of a pharmacy QA program is to promote medication safety by _____.
   a. reducing errors
   b. increasing performance
   c. improving processes and systems
   d. All of the above

7. Transcription and verification errors account for _____ percent of medication errors that occur at this stage of the medication use process.
   a. 11
   b. 12
   c. 38
   d. 39

8. Dispensing errors account for _____ percent of medication errors that occur at this stage of the medication use process.
   a. 11
   b. 12
   c. 38
   d. 39

9. The most useful methodology for initiating a CQI project is the use of _____.
   a. Deming or Stewarts, also called FOCUS-PDCA cycle
   b. root cause analysis (RCA)
   c. failure mode and effects analysis (FMEA)
   d. All of the above

10. This step of the FOCUS quality improvement process involves collecting data regarding the process by using data collection tools such as a flowchart of the current procedure and then determining where the variances lie.
    a. Find
    b. Understand
    c. Select
    d. Clarify

CRITICAL THINKING

Based on what you have learned in the textbook, answer the following questions.

1. You are a new pharmacy technician at the corner pharmacy and have noticed that many of the current pharmacy technicians are not asking open-ended questions to the patients when picking up their prescriptions. Knowing that this step in the medication use process is important to help prevent medication errors, how can you lead the pharmacy always to ask these types of questions when patients pick up their prescriptions?

_____

_____

_____

2. To prevent distribution errors in the pharmacy, all pharmacy staff should be careful not to dispense outdated or expired medications. Using the PDCA cycle described in the chapter, outline how you could help your pharmacy keep up with outdated or expired medication on the pharmacy shelves.

_____

_____

_____

INTERNET EXERCISES

Answer the following questions by researching your answers on the Internet.

1. With medication errors on the rise, a quality and safety leader should be in place in every pharmacy who can help focus on redesigning the system to make it resistant to errors. Research resources that are available specifically to the profession of pharmacy to help train and develop a medication safety leader for the pharmacy.

_____

_____

_____

2. Research the PPMI Summit and advancing the use of pharmacy technicians. If the beliefs and assumptions discussed at the PPMI Summit for pharmacy technician practice are brought to fruition, how can the leadership role of pharmacy technicians change?

_____

_____

_____

23 Certification Review for Pharmacy Technicians

KEY TERMINOLOGY

Provide a definition for each term.

1. Certification:

   _____

   _____

2. Licensure:

   _____

   _____

3. Registration:

   _____

   _____

FILL IN THE BLANK

Complete each statement by providing the word(s) missing where the blank is shown.

1. Most states regulate the pharmacy technician practice by requiring some type of prerequisite knowledge or _____ _____ to work in the field.

2. Each state has a regulating body known as the _____ _____ _____.

3. The licensing process ensures employers that each pharmacy technician has completed _____ _____ before his or her initial licensure.

4. Some state boards of pharmacy require that the license certificate be displayed in the pharmacy where an individual is _____.

5. If a particular state requires pharmacy technicians to be licensed, the license must be kept _____ in order for the pharmacy technician to remain eligible to work.

6. Often there is a requirement to complete a certain number of _____ _____ credits to be eligible for (license) renewal.

7. As with licensure, registration must be kept current and usually is renewed either _____ or _____.

8. A _____ certified pharmacy technician is one who successfully passes either of the two examinations: PTCE or ExCPT.

9. _____ also demonstrates to the public that the individual pharmacy technician has attained the necessary level of knowledge, skill, and experience in the field.

10. Certification of pharmacy technicians assists pharmacists and state boards of pharmacy by upholding _____ _____ standards to protect public safety.

MATCHING

Match each pharmacy technician certification examination with its corresponding description.

1. _____ Multiple-choice layout with four possible answers

2. _____ Administered by the Pharmacy Technician Certification Board (PTCB)

3. _____ Applicant must achieve a score of 650 points out of 900 possible points to pass successfully

4. _____ Consists of 90 questions

5. _____ Administered as part of the National Health Center Association

6. _____ Has a 2-hour time limit

7. _____ Consists of 110 questions

8. _____ Drugs and drug products comprise 23% of the examination

9. _____ Assisting the pharmacist in serving patients is 66% of the examination

10. _____ Applicant must achieve a score of 390 points out of 500 possible points to pass

a. PTCE

b. ExCPT

c. Both PTCE and ExCPT

MULTIPLE CHOICE

Select the best answer for each question.

1. _____ has the authority to write regulations and rules that pertain to all pharmacies within a particular state and is also in charge of issuing licenses for each pharmacy and pharmacist according to the state regulations.
   a. Food and Drug Administration
   b. State Board of Pharmacy
   c. Drug Enforcement Agency
   d. American Society of Health-System Pharmacists

2. Requirements to obtain a pharmacy technician license may include _____.
   a. proof of a high school diploma or a general education development (GED) certificate
   b. completion of a pharmacy technician training program
   c. successful passing of a national certification examination
   d. All of the above

3. Some states also require the submission of _____ as part of the background check process when applying for a pharmacy technician license.
   a. drug test
   b. college credit
   c. fingerprints
   d. hair sample

4. Individuals with a criminal history related to theft, drug use, or _____ may be disallowed from gaining registration.
   a. drug distribution
   b. DWI
   c. public intoxication
   d. indecency

5. Misdemeanor offenses are generally evaluated and investigated on a case-by-case basis by state board compliance officers and would include _____.
   a. driving under the influence (DUI)
   b. public intoxication
   c. driving while intoxicated (DWI)
   d. All of the above

6. The _____ is a professional organization that oversees the state boards of pharmacy.
   a. ASHP
   b. ACPE
   c. NABP
   d. FDA

7. To register as a pharmacy technician, in addition to an application fee, an applicant may be required to _____.
   a. show proof of a high school diploma or GED certificate
   b. provide proof of satisfactory work experience as a pharmacy technician
   c. complete a pharmacy technician training course or program
   d. All of the above

8. Once pharmacy technicians are certified, they are able to add the credentials _____ to the end of their name.
   a. PTCB
   b. CPhT
   c. ExCPT
   d. CPT

9. Which of the following would be a benefit to becoming a certified pharmacy technician?
   a. Demonstrates to the public that the individual pharmacy technician has attained the necessary level of knowledge, skill, and experience in the field
   b. Can help advance patient care and safety
   c. Helps uphold a high quality standard
   d. All of the above

10. After gaining the certified pharmacy technician credential, _____ hours of continuing education must be completed every 2 years to keep the certification active.
    a. 10
    b. 15
    c. 20
    d. 25

CRITICAL THINKING

Based on what you have learned in the textbook, answer the following questions.

1. Gentamicin is available as a pediatric 20 mg/2 mL IV solution. For all pediatric gentamicin IV orders, your hospital standard is to dilute to a concentration of 6 mg/mL. If you want to make 10 mL of the diluted concentration, how much gentamicin 20 mg/2 mL will you need, and how much diluent will you need?

_____

_____

_____

2. Vancomycin is available as a 1-g vial for IV administration. You will first need to reconstitute this medication to 100 mg/mL. How much diluent will you add? You will then need to dilute to 5 mg/mL for pediatric doses, 100 mL. How much vancomycin 100 mg/mL will you need, and how much diluent will you need?

_____

_____

_____

3. The first two questions of this section are examples of math calculations you may see on the pharmacy technician certification examination and may need to perform while working as a pharmacy technician. Not knowing how to perform those calculations is detrimental to patient safety. While most states do not require certification for pharmacy technicians, what would be the benefit of obtaining certification besides knowing how to calculate medication doses such as the ones mentioned?

_____

_____

_____

INTERNET EXERCISES

Answer the following questions by researching your answers on the Internet.

1. Research the requirements of your individual state board of pharmacy to practice being a pharmacy technician in your state.

   _____

   _____

   _____

2. After obtaining the certified pharmacy technician credential, you must complete continuing education every 2 years to maintain the certification. Research pharmacy continuing education providers.

   _____

   _____

   _____

Printed and bound by CPI Group (UK) Ltd, Croydon, CR0 4YY

03/10/2024

01040310-0017